Clinical anatomy MCQs

Roger Dalton

Published by KAIRD press 2012

All contents are copyright © Roger Dalton

Contents

ABOUT THE AUTHOR.. 4
FOREWARD..5
ABDOMEN QUESTIONS...8
THORAX QUESTIONS..22
LOWER LIMB QUESTIONS..35
HEAD AND NECK QUESTIONS...39
SPINE QUESTIONS..56
ABDOMEN ANSWERS...62
THORAX ANSWERS..87
UPPER LIMB ANSWERS...95
LOWER LIMB ANSWERS..110
HEAD AND NECK ANSWERS..129
SPINE ANSWERS...158

About the author

Roger Dalton is a Consultant in Emergency Medicine at the Northern General Hospital, Sheffield, UK. He is the founder and course director of the Sheffield Emergency Medicine MCEM OSCE course, co-founder of MCEM International and co-founder of the Central FCEM course.

Information about the above courses can be found at:
www.sheffieldem.co.uk
www.mceminternational.com
www.centralfcem.com

Foreward

This MCQ book is based on the College of Emergency Medicine anatomy curriculum for MCEM part A. The questions reflect the aspects of anatomy that are relevant to 'shop floor' work in Emergency Departments.
It will also be of use to medical students and doctors training in surgery, anaesthesia and medicine.

The book is divided into 2 main sections, questions and answers. The questions are divided into sections reflecting areas of the body e.g. abdomen, thorax etc. The answers are similarly divided and have extensive explanatory notes accompanying the answers.

Each question has 4 stems. Each stem is either true or false i.e. within each question there may be 4 true answers, 4 false answers, or a combination of true and false answers.

I welcome any comments, please feel free to email me at admin@sheffieldem.co.uk.

Roger Dalton
November 2012

Questions

ABDOMEN QUESTIONS

1. Internal oblique: (T/F)
a) Inserts into the lower ribs
b) Contributes to rotation of the vertebral column
c) Is innervated by the iliohypogastric nerve
d) Originates from the iliac crest

2. Regarding ovarian pathology: (T/F)
a) Pain originating from the ovary can be referred to the medial thigh
b) Pain originating from the ovary can be referred to the flank and loin
c) Inguinal lymphadenopathy is not a feature of ovarian pathology
d) The ovary can be positioned in the pouch of Douglas

3. Porto-systemic anastomoses can be found: (T/F)
a) At the upper 1/3 of the oesophagus
b) Halfway down the anal canal
c) In the paraumbilical veins
d) In the retroperitoneum

4. Regarding the pelvic ligaments: (T/F)
a) The sacrotuberous membrane runs from the lateral aspect of the sacrum to the iliac crest
b) The sacrospinous ligament runs from the lateral part of the sacrum to the spine of the ischium
c) The iliolumbar ligament runs from the spinous process of the 5th lumbar vertebra to the iliac crest
d) The sacrococcygeal joint is immobile

5. The rectus sheath: (T/F)
a) Is formed by the aponeurosis of rectus abdominis
b) Has the linea alba in the midline
c) Has the peritoneum directly deep to it
d) Has pyramidalis lying superficially to it

6. The pancreas: (T/F)
a) Produces glucagon from the beta cells
b) Crosses the midline
c) Lies on the transpyloric plane
d) Produces pancreatic lipase from the delta cells of the Islets of Langerhans

7. The inferior epigastric artery: (T/F)
a) Is a branch of the internal iliac artery
b) Runs between the rectus sheath and rectus abdominis
c) Anastomoses with intercostal arteries
d) Is related to the broad ligament at its origin

8. Regarding the blood supply of the liver: (T/F)
a) The hepatic artery gives off the right and left hepatic arteries after it has entered the liver
b) The portal vein divides into right and left branches in the porta hepatis, prior to entering the liver
c) The hepatic veins drain directly into the inferior vena cava
d) The portal vein is formed by the union of the inferior mesenteric vein and the splenic vein

9. Regarding the inguinal ligament: (T/F)
a) It runs from the anterior superior iliac spine to the pubic tubercle
b) It is comprised of the inferior border of the internal oblique aponeurosis
c) It lies above the spermatic cord
d) It becomes continuous with the fascia lata in the thigh

10. Regarding the male urethra: (T/F)
a) The widest part of the urethra is the membranous urethra
b) The narrowest part of the urethra is the membranous urethra
c) The external opening of the urethra at the glans is the narrowest part of the urethra
d) The urethra passes through the corpus spongiosum of the penis

11. The floor of the inguinal ligament is comprised of the following: (T/F)
a) The inguinal ligament
b) The lacunar ligament
c) The transversalis fascia
d) The conjoint tendon

12. Meckel's diverticulum: (T/F)
a) Arises from the distal jejunum
b) Is in close proximity to the iliocaecal valve
c) Is the remnant of the vitelline duct
d) Has an average length of 10cm

13. The testicular artery: (T/F)
a) Is a branch of the abdominal aorta
b) Gives a supply to the ureter
c) Passes through the superficial inguinal ring
d) Originates from the supra-renal aorta

14. The peritoneum: (T/F)
a) Is a 2 layered structure
b) Is a non-serous membrane
c) Contains the whole of the small bowel
d) Is a selectively permeable membrane

15. The transverse mesocolon: (T/F)
a) Connects the transverse colon to the liver
b) Contains the middle colic vessels
c) Is continuous with the lesser omentum
d) Separates the supracolic and the infracolic components

16. The superficial inguinal ring: (T/F)
a) Is a defect in the aponeurosis of internal oblique
b) Has the crest of the pubis below it
c) Has the spermatic cord passing through it
d) Has the iliohypogastric nerve passing through it

17. The kidneys: (T/F)
a) Are retroperitoneal
b) Are enclosed in a capsule
c) Have no exterior fascia
d) Move inferiorly by 2 to 2.5 cm during respiration

18. Regarding the infracolic compartment: (T/F)
a) It is divided into the right and left infracolic compartments by the small intestinal mesentery
b) Receptors within the small bowel mesentery can cause hypotension in the absence of haemorrhage
c) The right infracolic space is larger than the left
d) The left ureter crosses the border between the right and left infracolic compartments

19. Contents of the inguinal canal include: (T/F)
a) The spermatic cord
b) The broad ligament
c) The iliohypogastric nerve
d) The aponeurosis of external oblique

20. Concerning the greater omentum: (T/F)
a) It has a blood supply from a branch of the coeliac trunk
b) Its content of adipose tissue is not increased in obese people
c) It contributes to the immune system
d) It is attached to the lesser curve of the stomach

21. Regarding renal pathology: (T/F)
a) A perirenal abscess involves spread of pus into the retroperitoneal space
b) 'Renal pain' is felt in the T12 dermatome
c) Ureteric colic causes pain to be felt in the T11 and T12 dermatomes only
d) Flank pain is not a feature of renal infarction

22. Regarding the oesophagus: (T/F)
a) The cardiac orifice is at the level of the 12th thoracic vertebra
b) It is supplied by the vagus nerve
c) The posterior aspect of the abdominal oesophagus is covered with peritoneum
d) It has a blood supply derived from the abdominal aorta

23. The following are contents of the spermatic cord: (T/F)
a) Testicular artery
b) Genitofemoral nerve
c) Ilioinguinal nerve
d) Pampiniform plexus

24. Regarding the liver: (T/F)
a) The liver is the largest organ in the human body
b) The right and left lobes are separated by the ligamentum teres
c) The left lobe is larger than the right lobe
d) It is completely covered by peritoneum

25. Regarding the stomach: (T/F)
a) The fundus is located inferiorly to the cardiac orifice
b) The lesser curvature gives attachment to the hepatogastric ligament
c) The pyloric antrum secretes somatostatin and insulin
d) The pyloric sphincter has a layer of striated muscle

26. External oblique: (T/F)
a) Originates from the lower eight ribs
b) Forms the superior wall (roof) of the inguinal canal
c) Forms the linea alba in the midline
d) Inserts into the iliac crest

27. The nerve supply of the stomach: (T/F)
a) Is derived from the vagus nerve
b) Has separate branches to the anterior and posterior aspects
c) Is derived from the coeliac plexus
d) Is contained within the submucosa

28. The porta hepatis: (T/F)
a) Is on the posterior surface of the liver
b) Has no attachment to the omentum
c) Contains the portal vein
d) Contains the hepatic ducts

29. Scarpa's fascia: (T/F)
a) Is deep to the external oblique muscle
b) Is adherent to the linea alba
c) Descends to the scrotum
d) Is thicker than the superficial fascia

30. Regarding the duodenum: (T/F)
a) It has a blood supply derived from the superior mesenteric artery
b) It has a blood supply derived from the hepatic artery
c) Its venous drainage is to the inferior mesenteric vein
d) The head of the pancreas lies on the transpyloric plane

31. The vermiform appendix: (T/F)
a) Arises from the base of the caecum
b) Derives its blood supply from the inferior mesenteric artery
c) Is always intraperitoneal
d) Does not have a muscular layer

32. The ascending colon: (T/F)
a) Is retroperitoneal
b) Passes medially to the gallbladder below the liver
c) Is supplied by a branch of the superior mesenteric artery
d) Has the inferolateral aspect of the right kidney posterior to it as it ascends to the hepatic flexure

33. The duodenum: (T/F)
a) Is the longest part of the small intestine
b) Is entirely covered by mesentery
c) Has the head of the pancreas posterior and inferior to its first part
d) Has the aorta posterior to its third part

34. Regarding the inferior vena cava: (T/F)
a) It has a variable number of anterior visceral tributaries
b) It receives 2 suprarenal veins
c) It receives the renal veins at the level of the L1 vertebra
d) It receives the left testicular vein directly

35. The sigmoid colon: (T/F)
a) Becomes continuous with the rectum anterior to the 3rd sacral vertebra
b) Is supplied by branches of the iliac arteries
c) Is completely covered by peritoneum
d) Receives parasympathetic supply directly from the vagus nerve

36. Regarding the abdominal aorta: (T/F)
a) It gives off 4 lateral visceral branches
b) It gives off 5 lateral abdominal branches
c) It has 2 terminal branches
d) It has 3 anterior visceral branches

37. The following are part of the direct arterial supply to the stomach: (T/F)
a) Left gastric artery
b) Hepatic artery
c) Splenic artery
d) Right gastroepiploic artery

38. Regarding the biliary ducts: (T/F)
a) The common hepatic duct is formed by union of the right and left hepatic ducts only
b) The common bile duct runs through the greater omentum
c) The common bile duct forms the ampulla of Vater when it is joined by the pancreatic duct
d) The ampulla of Vater is surrounded by a circular layer of smooth muscle

39. The transverse colon: (T/F)
a) Is the least mobile part of the colon
b) Is connected to the pancreas and the posterior abdominal wall by the transverse mesocolon
c) Is supplied by the middle colic artery
d) Runs anterior to the greater curvature of the stomach

40. Regarding the liver: (T/F)
a) The left lobe is divided into the caudate lobe and the quadrate lobe
b) The gallbladder is the only structure that forms the division between the caudate and quadrate lobes
c) The fissure containing the ligamentum teres lies between the left lobe and the quadrate lobe
d) The fissure for the ligamentum venosum lies between the left lobe and the caudate lobe

41. The descending colon: (T/F)
a) Descends between psoas major and quadratus lumborum
b) Lies lateral to the right kidney
c) Is supplied by branches of the superior mesenteric artery
d) Has its venous drainage directly into the inferior vena cava

42. The jejunum: (T/F)
a) Does not have a mesenteric attachment
b) Has a wider lumen than the ileum
c) Derives its blood supply from the superior mesenteric artery
d) Can be a cause of referred pain in the T9/T10 dermatomes

43. Regarding the liver: (T/F)
a) The coronary ligament attaches the liver to the greater omentum
b) The coronary ligament is comprised of 2 reflected layers of visceral peritoneum
c) The bare area of the liver is the area which has no peritoneal covering
d) The bare area is not covered by the fibrous liver capsule

44. Regarding the lumbar plexus: (T/F)
a) It is formed by the 1st to 5th lumbar nerves
b) It is situated within the psoas muscle
c) The femoral nerve arises from the lumbar plexus
d) The nerve to the quadratus femoris arises from the lumbar plexus

45. Regarding the triangular ligaments: (T/F)
a) The right triangular ligament is formed by the layers of the coronary ligament
b) The right triangular ligament connects the liver to the diaphragm
c) The left triangular ligament is continuous with the coronary ligament
d) The left triangular ligament connects the liver to the diaphragm

46. The gallbladder: (T/F)
a) Has an arterial blood supply from the left hepatic artery
b) Contracts in response to a hormone produced in the duodenum
c) Is continuous with the cystic duct
d) Is separated from the liver by a layer of peritoneum

47. Regarding the portal vein: (T/F)
a) It is formed by the union of the superior mesenteric vein and the splenic vein
b) It drains blood from the spleen
c) It drains blood from the bile ducts
d) It drains blood from the pancreas

48. The testicles: (T/F)
a) Have their lymphatic drainage to the para-aortic nodes
b) Drain directly to the inferior vena cava
c) Descend in utero through the inguinal canal
d) Can survive for 24 hours following testicular torsion

49. The pancreas: (T/F)
a) Derives its blood supply from the splenic artery
b) Has its venous drainage directly into the portal vein
c) Is associated with referred pain to the T6 to T10 dermatomes
d) Is situated within the peritoneum

50. The spleen: (T/F)
a) Is not surrounded by peritoneum
b) Is retroperitoneal
c) Is supplied by a branch of the superior mesenteric artery
d) Has its venous drainage into the portal system

51. The abdominal aorta: (T/F)
a) Enters the abdomen through the diaphragm at the level of the T10 vertebra
b) Divides into the common iliac arteries at the level of the 4th lumbar vertebra
c) Gives off the renal artery as its first branch
d) Descends anterior to the lumbar vertebral bodies

52. Regarding the surface of the liver: (T/F)
a) The groove for the inferior vena cava lies between the right and left lobes
b) The fossa containing the gallbladder lies between the right lobe and the caudate lobe
c) The area between the gallbladder and the liver is covered with peritoneum
d) The hepatic veins join the inferior vena cava adjacent to the junction of the right lobe and the caudate lobe

53. The inferior vena cava: (T/F)
a) Is formed by the union of the iliac and femoral veins
b) Is formed at the level of the L4 vertebra
c) Ascends on the left side of the vertebral column
d) Enters the diaphragm at the level of the T8 vertebra

54. Regarding gallbladder pathology: (T/F)
a) Gallstones are frequently asymptomatic
b) Shoulder tip pain indicates irritation of the sub-diaphragmatic peritoneum
c) Biliary colic is always related to the presence of gallstones
d) Cholangitis is inflammation of the gallbladder

55. Regarding the kidneys: (T/F)
a) They have no external fat
b) The lymphatic drainage of the kidneys is into the para-aortic nodes
c) The left kidney is lower than the right
d) They are palpable in normal, healthy individuals

56. Regarding the bladder: (T/F)
a) The apex points superiorly
b) The base faces inferiorly
c) The neck of the bladder points inferiorly
d) The superior surface is covered with peritoneum

57. The following structures can be palpated on a rectal examination in a healthy individual: (T/F)
a) The rectovesical pouch
b) The prostate gland
c) The ovary
d) The cervix

58. Regarding the prostate gland: (T/F)
a) It is not surrounded by a capsule
b) The base of the prostate is adjacent to the femoral neck
c) It is a lobular structure
d) It has its lymphatic drainage to the internal iliac nodes

59. The supracolic compartment contains: (T/F)
a) Stomach
b) Liver
c) Kidneys
d) Spleen

60. The ovaries: (T/F)
a) Are attached to the broad ligament
b) Receive their blood supply via the round ligament
c) Receive their blood supply from a direct branch of the abdominal aorta
d) Drain directly into the inferior vena cava bilaterally

61. Regarding the sacral plexus: (T/F)
a) It is formed by the 4th and 5th lumbar and 1st to 4th sacral nerves
b) The sciatic nerve arises from the sacral plexus
c) The pudendal nerve is derived from the L4 and L5 nerves
d) The sciatic nerve exits the pelvis via the obturator foramen

62. The bladder: (T/F)
a) In adults, is pyramidal in shape when empty
b) Becomes circular in shape as it fills
c) In children, drops down into the pelvis as it fills
d) In adults, displaces the rectum to expand posteriorly as it fills

63. Regarding prostate cancer: (T/F)
a) It is an adenocarcinoma
b) Tumour staging involves the number of prostate lobes involved
c) It can spread locally into the rectum
d) It rarely metastases to bone

64. The infracolic compartment contains: (T/F)
a) Small bowel
b) Descending colon
c) Bladder
d) Ascending colon

65. Regarding the spleen: (T/F)
a) It is essential for life
b) It lies under the 7th to 9th ribs
c) It is visible on FAST ultrasound
d) It has a notched posterior border

THORAX QUESTIONS

1. Regarding the dermatomes of the anterior thoracic wall: (T/F)
a) The nipples are within the T4 dermatome
b) The nipples are within the T6 dermatome
c) The umbilicus lies at the T12 dermatome
d) The umbilicus lies at the level of the T10 dermatome

2. Regarding the intercostal muscles: (T/F)
a) There are 12 sets (right and left) of external intercostal muscles
b) There are 11 sets of internal intercostal muscles
c) The innermost intercostal muscles contain the intercostal neurovascular bundle
d) The transversus thoracus muscle arises from the sternum

3. Regarding the diaphragm: (T/F)
a) The opening for the inferior vena cava is at the level of T10
b) The opening for the oesophagus is at the level of T10
c) It is solely innervated by the phrenic nerve
d) A hiatus hernia involves the abdominal oesophagus rising through the oesophageal opening

4. Regarding the diaphragm: (T/F)
a) Paralysis at the level of C4 will have no effect on diaphragmatic function
b) The opening for the aorta is at the level of T10
c) Congenital hernias of the diaphragm are mostly left sided
d) The diaphragm relaxes during inhalation

5. During a 'clamshell' thoracotomy: (T/F)
a) The internal mammary arteries are not at risk of being damaged
b) A Gigli saw is used to cut through the ribs
c) The superior part of the mediastinum is easily reached
d) The chest cannot always be surgically closed following a clamshell thoracotomy

6. The thoracic inlet: (T/F)
a) Has the 1st thoracic vertebrae posteriorly
b) Has the costal cartilage of the first rib and the superior border of the manubrium anteriorly
c) Transmits the trachea
d) Transmits the phrenic nerve

7. The trachea: (T/F)
a) Commences at the level of the 6th cervical vertebrae
b) Has the recurrent laryngeal nerves posterior to it
c) Is reinforced with cartilaginous rings posteriorly and laterally
d) Lies in the superior mediastinum in the thorax

8. The thymus: (T/F)
a) Has the 5th costal cartilage as its lower border
b) Extends upwards to the lower border of the thyroid
c) Is at its largest during childhood
d) Normally consists of a heterogenous mass

9. Regarding the heart valves: (T/F)
a) The mitral valve has 3 leaflets
b) The closing of the mitral valve and the tricuspid valve constitutes the first heart sound
c) The aortic valve has 2 leaflets
d) The pulmonary valve has 2 leaflets

10. Regarding the pericardium: (T/F)
a) The serous pericardium has 2 layers
b) The phrenic nerve runs over its surface
c) It is supplied by a branch of the external mammary artery
d) It has a potential space between the fibrous and serous layers

11. Regarding the great vessels: (T/F)
a) The aorta gives off the right and left coronary arteries as it leaves the left ventricle
b) The superior vena cava is separated from the right atrium by a valve
c) The pulmonary artery is the only artery in humans to carry de-oxygenated blood
d) The inferior vena cava is retroperitoneal

12. The oesophagus: (T/F)
a) Begins at the level of the C6 vertebrae
b) Ends at the level of the T12 vertebrae
c) Passes posterior to the left main bronchus
d) Passes through the diaphragm at the level of the T10 vertebra

13. The oesophagus has specific areas of constriction which are located: (T/F)
a) Where it is crossed by the thyroid gland
b) Behind the cricoid cartilage
c) Where its anterior surface is crossed by the aortic arch
d) Where it pierces the diaphragm

14. Regarding the lungs: (T/F)
a) The left lung has 3 lobes
b) The right lung has 3 lobes
c) The horizontal fissure lies anteriorly at the level of the 4th costal cartilage
d) The oblique fissure lies anteriorly at the level of the 4th costal cartilage

15. Regarding thoracic injuries: (T/F)
a) A flail chest is defined as a single rib, fractured in 2 places
b) Pulmonary contusion is rare in a flail chest injury
c) Rupture of the right diaphragm is more common than rupture of the left
d) Sternal fracture may be associated with myocardial contusion

16. The azygos vein: (T/F)
a) Has the pericardial veins draining into it
b) Is the continuation of the left ascending lumbar vein
c) Runs up the right side of the thoracic vertebral column
d) Enters the diaphragm at the level of T10

17. Regarding the ribs: (T/F)
a) The upper 6 ribs are attached directly to the sternum
b) All the ribs are attached to the thoracic vertebrae
c) The lowest 2 ribs are 'floating ribs'
d) The 1st rib articulates with the body of the sternum

18. Regarding the pleura: (T/F)
a) It has 2 layers
b) The pleural cavity contains no fluid in healthy individuals
c) The visceral pleura is highly sensitive to pain
d) Mesothelioma affects the pleura rather than lung parenchyma

19. The sinoatrial node: (T/F)
a) Is receptive to sympathetic innervation only
b) Normally has an arterial supply arising from the right coronary artery
c) Lies near the entrance of the superior vena cava to the heart
d) Normally has a pacemaker action setting the heart rate at 60 to 100 beats per minute

20. Regarding heart sounds: (T/F)
a) The 1st heart sound is related to the closure of the aortic and pulmonary valves
b) The 2nd heart sound is related to the closure of the aortic and pulmonary valves
c) A split 2nd heart sound can occur in healthy individuals
d) A grade 6 heart murmur requires a stethoscope to hear it

UPPER LIMB QUESTIONS

1. Regarding shoulder dislocations: (T/F)
a) Luxio erectae is a type of posterior shoulder dislocation
b) Posterior shoulder dislocation is associated with epileptic seizures
c) Anterior shoulder dislocation is associated with permanent axillary nerve injury
d) Posterior shoulder dislocation rarely has a delay in diagnosis

2. The origins of Pectoralis major include: (T/F)
a) The posterior surface of the sternal half of the clavicle
b) The anterior surface of the sternum
c) The aponeurosis of the external oblique muscle
d) The cartilages of the 'true ribs'

3. The ulnar nerve: (T/F)
a) Arises from the medial cord of the brachial plexus
b) Supplies the 1st and 2nd lumbrical muscles
c) Innervates all the interossei muscles
d) Is involved in Erb's palsy

4. De Quervain's tenosynovitis: (T/F)
a) Involves the tendon of extensor pollicis longus
b) Involves the tendon of abductor pollicis longus
c) Finkelstein's test is part of the standard examination
d) Surgery is needed in most cases

5. Teres major: (T/F)
a) Is a lateral rotator of the humerus
b) It contributes to extension of the arm at the shoulder
c) It is supplied by the superior subscapular nerve
d) It inserts into the medial lip of the bicipital groove of the humerus

6. The lumbricals: (T/F)
a) Extend the metacarpophalangeal joints
b) Flex the metacarpophalangeal joints
c) Extend the interphalangeal joints
d) Flex the interphalangeal joints

7. Regarding serratus anterior: (T/F)
a) It inserts into the lateral border of the scapula
b) Its origin is the upper 8 or 9 ribs
c) It is supplied in part by the medial thoracic artery
d) It is supplied by the long thoracic nerve

8. The acromioclavicular joint: (T/F)
a) Derives its stability from 4 ligaments
b) Is a synovial joint
c) A grade 3 dislocation of the AC joint involves disruption of the acromioclavicular and coracoclavicular ligaments
d) Subacromial impingement rarely involves night pain, waking the patient from sleep

9. The brachial plexus: (T/F)
a) Has 6 roots
b) Has 3 trunks
c) Has 6 divisions
d) Has 4 cords

10. Opponens pollicis: (T/F)
a) Is supplied by the ulnar nerve
b) Lies medial to flexor pollicis brevis
c) Inserts into the base of the thumb metacarpal only
d) Originates in part from the flexor retinaculum

11. Regarding the scapula: (T/F)
a) Scapular fracture can be regarded as a 'minor injury'
b) Winging of the scapula is commonly caused by serratus anterior palsy
c) It is stationary during movements of the shoulder
d) The superior border of the scapula is palpable

12. The biceps: (T/F)
a) Are supplied by the brachial artery
b) Are innervated by the brachial nerve
c) The brachial pulse is palpated laterally to the biceps tendon
d) Tears of the short head of biceps are more common than tears of the long head

13. The 'triangle of safety' is bounded by the following: (T/F)
a) Anterior border of latissimus dorsi
b) Anterior border of serratus anterior
c) Lateral border of the pectoralis major muscle
d) 5th intercostal space

14. The brachial artery: (T/F)
a) Is the continuation of the axillary artery commencing at the upper border of teres major
b) Has only the radial artery as a terminal branch
c) Lies deep at the elbow
d) Lies lateral to the median nerve in the cubital fossa

15. The median nerve: (T/F)
a) Is the only nerve running through the carpal tunnel
b) Injury at the wrist would result in a 'clawed hand'
c) Supplies all the flexor muscles of the forearm
d) Injury to the median nerve causes loss of thumb opposition

16. Regarding supraspinatus: (T/F)
a) It originates from the spine of the scapula
b) It is innervated by the superior subscapular nerve
c) It is supplied by the suprascapular artery
d) It is a rotator of the humerus

17. Regarding the triceps: (T/F)
a) All 3 heads originate from the posterior humerus
b) They are innervated by the radial nerve
c) Their only action is extension at the elbow
d) They are supplied by a branch of the brachial artery

18. The radial nerve: (T/F)
a) Has no sensory supply to the hand
b) It arises from the roots of C5 to T1
c) Radial nerve damage can cause wrist drop
d) Atraumatic radial nerve damage is always permanent

19. The medial epicondyle of the elbow: (T/F)
a) Is the common extensor origin
b) Has the ulnar nerve running anteriorly
c) Is inflammed in 'tennis elbow'
d) Ossification of the medial epicondyle begins before the lateral epicondyle

20. The axillary nerve: (T/F)
a) When damaged, causes problems with shoulder adduction
b) Directly supplies the skin overlying the deltoid
c) Lies in the triangular space
d) Contributes to the innervation of triceps

21. Flexor carpi ulnaris: (T/F)
a) Originates exclusively from the medial epicondyle
b) Inserts to the distal ulna
c) The ulnar artery is medial to flexor carpi ulnaris at the wrist
d) Is supplied by the ulnar nerve

22. Flexor pollicis longus: (T/F)
a) Inserts to the base of the proximal phalanx of the thumb
b) The tendon of flexor pollicis longus runs through the carpal tunnel
c) It is innervated by the ulnar nerve
d) Has a role in wrist flexion

23. Flexor carpi radialis: (T/F)
a) Originates from the medial epicondyle
b) Inserts into the hook of the hamate
c) Is supplied by the radial nerve
d) Its action is limited to wrist flexion

24. The radial artery: (T/F)
a) Arises in the cubital fossa
b) Is the main contributor to the superficial palmar arch
c) Is easily palpable at the wrist in patients with a systolic blood pressure of less than 70mmHg
d) If damaged, can lead to aneurysm formation

25. The ulnar artery: (T/F)
a) Arises directly from the axillary artery
b) Patency can be checked by Neer's test
c) Terminates in the deep palmar arch
d) Lies deep to the flexor retinaculum

26. Brachialis: (T/F)
a) Is an extender of the elbow
b) Is supplied by the radial nerve
c) Contributes to pronation and supination
d) Isolated brachialis injuries are common

27. The lateral epicondyle of the elbow: (T/F)
a) Is the common extensor origin
b) Is inflamed in tennis elbow
c) Gives rise to the radial collateral ligament
d) Is the origin of pronator teres

28. Extensor digitorum: (T/F)
a) Arises from the lateral epicondyle of the humerus
b) Has insertions to all 5 digits
c) Its principle action is on the proximal phalanges
d) It is supplied by the anterior interosseous nerve

29. The cephalic vein: (T/F)
a) Lies medially in the arm
b) Communicates with the basilic vein
c) Is a good site for large bore venous cannulation
d) Drains into the basilic vein

30. The anatomical snuff box: (T/F)
a) Is bounded by the tendon of extensor pollicis brevis
b) Has the radial styloid as its proximal border
c) Has a blood supply which enters distally
d) Has the median nerve as one of its contents

31. The deltoid muscle: (T/F)
a) Is supplied by the axillary nerve
b) Its function can be damaged following breast surgery
c) It is supplied directly by the axillary artery
d) Is the main abductor of the humerus at the shoulder

32. Abductor pollicis brevis: (T/F)
a) Can be palpated in the thenar eminence
b) Is innervated by the ulnar nerve
c) Draws the thumb forward in a plane at right angles to that of the palm of the hand
d) Inserts into the base of the thumb metacarpal

33. The quadrangular space: (T/F)
a) Has teres major as one of its boundaries
b) Has the humerus as one of its boundaries
c) Contains the axillary artery
d) Can be damaged in posterior shoulder dislocations

34. The contents of the carpal tunnel include: (T/F)
a) The tendon of flexor digitorum profundus
b) The radial nerve
c) The tendon of flexor pollicis longus
d) The tendon of flexor digitorum superficialis

35. Regarding the interossei of the hand: (T/F)
a) There are 3 dorsal interossei
b) There are 3 palmar interossei
c) They are supplied by the ulnar nerve
d) The dorsal interossei abduct the fingers away from the middle finger

36. Regarding latissimus dorsi: (T/F)
a) It is supplied by a branch of the subscapular artery
b) It is an external rotator of the arm
c) It inserts into the humerus
d) It is supplied by a branch of the posterior cord of the brachial plexus

37. The ulnar nerve: (T/F)
a) Can be directly damaged following a fracture of the humerus
b) Runs through the carpal tunnel
c) Is medial to the ulnar artery at the wrist
d) Is derived from the posterior cord of the brachial plexus

38. Regarding trapezius: (T/F)
a) Its origin includes the nuchal ligament
b) It inserts into the wing of the scapula
c) Its innervation is via the dorsal rami of C3 and C4
d) It is innervated by a branch of the thyrocervical trunk

39. Regarding forearm fractures: (T/F)
a) A Monteggia fracture is a fracture of the ulna with dislocation of the radial head
b) A Galeazzi fracture a fracture of the ulna with dislocation of the distal radioulnar joint
c) A Barton's fracture is a distal radius fracture with dislocation of the radiocarpal joint
d) A Smith's fracture is a distal radius fracture with dorsal displacement of the distal fracture segment

40. Subscapularis: (T/F)
a) Arises from the subscapular fossa
b) Inserts into the greater tubercle of the humerus
c) Is supplied by branches of the lateral cord of the brachial plexus
d) It medially rotates the humerus

LOWER LIMB QUESTIONS

1. Flexor hallucis longus: (T/F)
a) Is a plantar flexor of the foot
b) Inserts into the base of the proximal phalanx of the great toe
c) Is supplied by the tibial nerve
d) Contributes to being able to stand on tip-toes

2. Sartorius: (T/F)
a) Is the longest muscle in the human body
b) Originates from the anterior superior iliac spine
c) Contributes to knee flexion
d) Is innervated by the sciatic nerve

3. Biceps femoris: (T/F)
a) Is an extender of the hip joint
b) Is innervated by branches of the sciatic nerve
c) Arises entirely within the pelvis
d) Inserts only into the fibula

4. The medial collateral ligament: (T/F)
a) Originates from the medial epicondyle of the femur
b) Inserts into the medial condyle of the tibia
c) Is characteristically damaged by a varus injury
d) Has a insertion into the medial meniscus

5. Regarding hip adduction: (T/F)
a) The majority of the hip adductors are supplied by the obturator nerve
b) The hip adductors originate from the pubic ramus and symphysis
c) The hip adductors are supplied by the L2 to L4 nerves
d) The obturator nerve has a sensory supply to the anterior thigh

6. Peroneus brevis: (T/F)
a) Is supplied by the tibial artery
b) Is a plantar flexor of the foot
c) Can cause an avulsion fracture of the base of the 5th metatarsal if over-stretched
d) Is supplied by the deep peroneal nerve

7. The femoral artery: (T/F)
a) Arises directly from the external iliac artery
b) The superficial femoral artery supplies the thigh
c) Contributes a supply to the genitals
d) Becomes the popliteal artery in the adductor hiatus

8. The great saphenous vein: (T/F)
a) Is visible over the lateral malleolus of the ankle
b) Drains into the external iliac vein
c) When thrombosed, constitutes a deep venous thrombosis
d) Is a common site of varicose veins

9. Regarding lymph nodes: (T/F)
a) The superficial inguinal lymph nodes are situated above the inguinal ligament
b) The node of Ranvier is found in the deep inguinal lymph nodes
c) The deep inguinal lymph nodes drain into the external iliac lymph nodes
d) The external iliac lymph nodes drain directly into the para-aortic lymph nodes

10. The following are components of the deltoid ligament of the ankle joint: (T/F)
a) Calcaneotibial ligament
b) Anterior talotibial
c) Posterior talocalcaneal ligament
d) Medial talocalcaneal ligament

11. Psoas major: (T/F)
a) Arises from the T12 to L5 vertebrae and their intervertebral discs
b) Inserts into the greater trochanter of the femur
c) Is a medial rotator of the thigh
d) Is innervated by the femoral nerve

12. The following bones are components of the lateral arch of the foot: (T/F)
a) Calcaneum
b) Cuboid
c) 3rd, 4th and 5th metatarsals
d) Lateral cuneiform

13. Regarding the anterior thigh: (T/F)
a) Iliacus is a medial hip rotator
b) Iliacus originates in part from the anterior superior iliac spine
c) Pectineus is a medial hip rotator
d) Pectineus can form the covering of an obturator hernia

14. The medial meniscus: (T/F)
a) Heals quickly after injury if the injury is to the inner part of the medial meniscus
b) If removed surgically (menisectomy), leads to a higher risk of osteoarthritis
c) If injured, is characteristically injured in isolation
d) Is not involved in the pattern of injury known as O'Donoghue's triad

15. Rectus Femoris: (T/F)
a) Inserts into the patella
b) Arises in part from the anterior superior iliac spine
c) Is supplied by the sciatic nerve
d) Is an extender of the knee

16. The dorsalis pedis artery: (T/F)
a) Is palpable medial to the tendon of extensor hallucis longus
b) Is always palpable in young healthy individuals
c) Is the continuation of the anterior tibial artery
d) Gives off the deep plantar artery

17. Damage to the common peroneal nerve: (T/F)
a) Can be caused by a Maisonneuve fracture
b) Can cause foot-drop
c) Can cause sensory loss on the dorsum of the foot
d) Can cause sensory loss over the heel

18. The following landmarks are components of the Ottawa ankle & foot rule: (T/F)
a) Lateral malleolus
b) Calcaneum
c) Navicular
d) Base of 5th metatarsal

19. Regarding lower limb compartment syndrome: (T/F)
a) Loss of peripheral pulses is an early sign
b) Pain is an early sign
c) It is always related to trauma
d) Rhabdomyolysis is a known consequence

20. The patellar tendon: (T/F)
a) Inserts into the tibia tuberosity
b) When inflamed, along with its insertion, is known as Kohler's syndrome
c) When ruptured, leads to an inability to straight leg raise
d) Has a bursa posterior to it

HEAD AND NECK QUESTIONS

1. Regarding sternocleidomastoid: (T/F)
a) It originates from the sternum only
b) It inserts into the occipital bone
c) Its only action is rotation of the head
d) Its anterior border covers the carotid arteries

2. The cricothyroid ligament: (T/F)
a) Forms the vocal ligaments
b) Can be located inferior to the thryoid cartilage
c) Receives the anterior end of each vocal cord
d) Receives the posterior end of each vocal cord

3. Horner's syndrome: (T/F)
a) Causes a dilated pupil
b) Is caused by a deficiency of sympathetic supply to the eye
c) Is associated with increased sweating
d) Causes total paralysis of the levator palpebrae superioris

4. Enlargement of the pituitary gland is associated with: (T/F)
a) Bilateral nasal visual field defects
b) Sheehan's syndrome
c) Erosion of the sella turcica
d) Headache

5. The glossopharyngeal nerve: (T/F)
a) Decends through the skull via the jugular foramen
b) Is entirely sensory
c) Contributes to blood pressure control
d) Supplies the posterior one-third of the tongue

6. The anterior triangle of the neck: (T/F)
a) Is bounded superiorly by the mandible
b) Is bounded anteriorly by the digastric muscle
c) Is bounded posteriorly by the sternocleidomastoid
d) Has the jugular notch of the manubrium as its apex

7. The medial wall of the orbit is formed by the following bones: (T/F)
a) Frontal process of the maxilla
b) Lacrimal bone
c) Greater wing of the sphenoid
d) Ethmoid

8. The thyroid gland: (T/F)
a) Has 4 lobes
b) Is directly supplied by the carotid artery
c) Has its venous drainage directly into the internal jugular vein
d) Has the parathyroid glands posterior to it

9. Regarding the facial vein: (T/F)
a) It communicates with the cavernous sinus
b) It is formed by the union of the superficial temporal and supraorbital veins
c) It drains into the external jugular vein
d) It crosses the face above the mandible as it descends

10. Clinical signs of a base of skull fracture include: (T/F)
a) Mastoid bruising
b) Blood in the external ear canal
c) Bleeding from the nostrils
d) Bilateral orbital ecchymoses

11. Regarding the carotid sheath: (T/F)
a) It is formed from prevertebral fascia only
b) It surrounds the external carotid artery
c) It surrounds the recurrent laryngeal nerve
d) It surrounds the vagus nerve

12. The oculomotor nerve: (T/F)
a) Enters the orbit through the superior orbital fissure
b) Supplies all the ocular muscles
c) Controls pupillary constriction
d) Runs along the medial wall of the cavernous sinus

13. Regarding scalenus anterior: (T/F)
a) It originates from the 3rd to 6th cervical vertebrae
b) It inserts into the medial clavicle
c) It is innervated by the C5 and C6 spinal nerves
d) It is a rotator of the neck

14. Clinical features of a middle cerebral artery stroke include the following: (T/F)
a) Ipsilateral hemiplegia
b) Eyes deviated toward the side of the infarction
c) Loss of consciousness
d) Contralateral hemianopia

15. The recurrent laryngeal nerve: (T/F)
a) Is a branch of the vagus nerve
b) On the right, runs around the subclavian artery
c) Supplies all the muscles of the larynx
d) If damaged, can cause a hoarse voice

16. The parotid gland contains: (T/F)
a) The facial nerve
b) The external carotid artery
c) The superficial temporal artery
d) The retromandibular vein

17. The temporal fossa (T/F)
a) Is entirely located over the temporal bone
b) Has the zygomatic arch inferior to it
c) Contains the superficial temporal artery
d) Contains the deep temporal nerves

18. The nasal cavity: (T/F)
a) Has 3 turbinates on each side
b) Is innervated by the trigeminal nerve
c) Has its blood supply from the maxillary artery only
d) The nasolacrimal duct drains into the middle meatus

19. The subclavian vein: (T/F)
a) Is the continuation of the axillary vein
b) Commences at the medial border of the clavicle
c) Contributes to the formation of the brachiocephalic vein
d) Has the thoracic duct draining into it on the right side

20. Regarding the facial nerve: (T/F)
a) It supplies taste fibres to the posterior third of the tongue
b) It supplies all the muscles of facial expression
c) It can be tested using the corneal reflex
d) It can be damaged by wounds in the pre-auricular area

21. Orbicularis oculi: (T/F)
a) Is supplied only by the temporal branch of the facial nerve
b) Closes the eyelids
c) Empties the lacrimal sac
d) Is not used in the corneal reflex

22. The pterygoid venous plexus: (T/F)
a) Communicates with the cavernous sinus
b) Is situated between the temporalis and medial pterygoid
c) Can be damaged during dental procedures
d) Communicates with the ophthalmic vein

23. Regarding the opthalmic division of the trigeminal nerve: (T/F)
a) The opthalmic nerve is a mixed motor and sensory nerve
b) The infratrochlear nerve supples the skin of the eyelids
c) The frontal nerve supplies the skin at the tip of the nose
d) The frontal nerve supplies the skin of the forehead and scalp

24. Buccinator: (T/F)
a) Arises entirely from the maxilla and mandible
b) Is supplied by the mandibular branch of the facial nerve
c) Pulls the angle of the mouth forwards
d) Inserts into the orbicularis oris

25. Regarding the branches of the external carotid artery: (T/F)
a) The facial artery supplies the tonsils
b) Injury to the middle meningeal artery classically results in a subdural haematoma
c) The maxillary artery is given off from the external carotid artery within the parotid gland
d) Branches of the occipital artery supplies the pinna

26. Regarding the submandibular lymph nodes: (T/F)
a) They receive lymph from the entire upper and lower lips
b) They receive lymph from the entire tongue
c) They receive lymph from the front of the scalp
d) They receive lymph from the facial sinuses

27. Occipitofrontalis: (T/F)
a) Has 2 bellies
b) Is innervated by the facial nerve
c) Originates in part from the frontal bone
d) Raises the eyebrow

28. Regarding the blood supply to the scalp: (T/F)
a) It is derived entirely from the external carotid artery
b) The posterior auricular artery supplies the pinna
c) The supraorbital artery does not supply the scalp
d) The superficial temporal artery is impalpable

29. Regarding the veins of the cranium and brain: (T/F)
a) They have no valves
b) They have thick walls
c) They drain to the venous sinuses
d) The diploic veins are situated in the cranial bones

30. Regarding the temporal bone: (T/F)
a) It has 5 bony components
b) The temporal line is located on the temporal bone
c) It has the ethmoid bone immediately anterior to it
d) It forms part of the temporal fossa

31. Masseter: (T/F)
a) Originates from the zygomatic arch
b) Is supplied by the facial nerve
c) Assists in chewing
d) Inserts into the body of the mandible

32. Regarding the parotid gland: (T/F)
a) It has 2 lobes
b) It is innervated by the facial nerve
c) Its duct passes between the masseter and buccinator
d) It is the smallest salivary gland

33. Regarding the maxillary division of the trigeminal nerve: (T/F)
a) The maxillary nerve is a mixed motor and sensory nerve
b) It supplies the skin on the side of the nose
c) The anterior superior alveolar nerve supplies the upper pre-molar teeth
d) The superior alveolar nerves supply the maxillary sinus

34. The infratemporal fossa: (T/F)
a) Is situated medial to the zygomatic arch
b) Contains the mandibular and maxillary nerves
c) Has the foramen rotundum within its borders
d) Has the medial pterygoid as its floor

35. The maxillary artery: (T/F)
a) Is a branch of the internal carotid artery
b) Gives off the middle meningeal artery
c) Supplies the pterygoids
d) Supplies the palate

36. Regarding the mandibular nerve: (T/F)
a) It is a division of the facial nerve
b) It is transmitted via the foramen ovale
c) It is entirely sensory
d) It has 3 divisions

37. Temporalis: (T/F)
a) Originates from the temporal fossa
b) Inserts into the mandible
c) Is innervated by the deep temporal nerves
d) Retracts the mandible

38. Regarding the branches of the trigeminal nerve: (T/F)
a) The auriculotemporal nerve supplies the external auditory meatus
b) The lingual nerve transmits taste fibres from the anterior 2/3 of the tongue
c) The inferior alveolar nerve supplies the skin of the chin
d) The buccal nerve supplies buccinator

39. The hypoglossal nerve: (T/F)
a) Is a mixed motor and sensory nerve
b) Descends through the skull via the jugular foramen
c) Supplies all the muscles of the tongue
d) Travels within the carotid sheath

40. The following are components of the roof of the nose: (T/F)
a) The body of the sphenoid
b) The nasal septum
c) The cribriform plate
d) The frontal bone

41. Regarding the mandibular division of the trigeminal nerve: (T/F)
a) The mandibular nerve is a mixed motor and sensory nerve
b) It supplies the anterior two-thirds of the tongue
c) It supplies the submandibular salivary glands
d) It supplies the parotid salivary gland

42. The external carotid artery: (T/F)
a) Begins at the level of the cricoid cartilage
b) Gives off the inferior thyroid artery
c) Runs superficial to platysma
d) Gives off the lingual artery

43. The arteries that anastomose in Little's area include: (T/F)
a) The posterior ethmoidal artery
b) The sphenopalatine artery
c) The greater palatine artery
d) The nasal artery

44. Regarding the teeth: (T/F)
a) There are 34 permanent teeth
b) The permanent incisors erupt at age 7 to 8 years
c) The deciduous molars erupt at age 6 to 8 months
d) The permanent canines erupt at age 11to 12 years

45. Regarding the adenoids and tonsils: (T/F)
a) The adenoids are situated in the oropharynx
b) The palatine tonsils are supplied by the lingual artery
c) Peritonsillar abscesses are usually bilateral
d) The tonsils drain to the superficial cervical chain of lymph nodes

46. Regarding the laryngeal cartilages: (T/F)
a) The cricoid cartilage is the largest of the laryngeal cartilages
b) The cricoid cartilage lies superior to the thyroid cartilage
c) The arytenoid cartilages have vocal processes
d) The corniculate cartilages are cone shaped

47. Regarding the larynx: (T/F)
a) The internal laryngeal nerve runs through the thyrohyoid membrane
b) The quadrangular membrane lies between the epiglottis and the thryoid cartilage
c) The digastric muscle attaches to the hyoid bone
d) The epiglottis is attached to the cricoid cartilage

48. Regarding the auditory ossicles: (T/F)
a) The malleus is the largest of the ossicles
b) The incus is attached to the oval window
c) The malleus is attached to the tympanic membrane
d) The tensor tympani muscle enhances transmission of sound from the tympanic membrane to the ossicles

49. Regarding the recurrent laryngeal nerve: (T/F)
a) Unilateral recurrent laryngeal nerve damage has no discernible clinical effect
b) Bilateral recurrent laryngeal nerve damage can result in airway compromise
c) It may be damaged in thyroid surgery
d) The right recurrent laryngeal nerve is longer than the left

50. Regarding the bony margins of the orbit: (T/F)
a) The roof of the orbit is formed by the frontal bone only
b) The lateral wall of the orbit is formed by the zygoma only
c) The floor of the orbit is formed by the maxilla only
d) The nasolacrimal canal is on the roof of the orbit

51. Regarding the eyelids: (T/F)
a) They contain a fibrous septum
b) The palpebral ligaments attach the tarsal plates to the orbit
c) The orbicularis oculi opens the eyes
d) The levator palpebrae superioris opens the eye

52. The accessory nerve: (T/F)
a) Is a mixed motor and sensory nerve
b) Descends through the skull via the jugular foramen
c) Innervates the pharynx
d) Supplies the sternocleidomastoid

53. Regarding the contents of the eye: (T/F)
a) The aqueous humor fills both the anterior and posterior chambers
b) The vitreous body is a pigmented gel
c) The lens is a bi-concave structure
d) The lens is attached to the ciliary body

54. Regarding the lacrimal apparatus: (T/F)
a) The lacrimal gland is supplied by the facial nerve
b) Tears enter the lacrimal sac via the canaliculi
c) The lacrimal gland lies on the medial wall of the orbit
d) The nasolacrimal duct enters the nose in the superior meatus

55. Regarding the extrinsic orbital muscles: (T/F)
a) Superior rectus raises the eye upwards
b) Lateral rectus rotates the eye to look outwards
c) Superior oblique is innervated by the abducent nerve
d) Inferior oblique is innervated by the oculomotor nerve

56. Regarding the auditory tube: (T/F)
a) The auditory tube links the middle ear to the oropharynx
b) The mastoid antrum connects to the inner ear
c) The mastoid air cells are continuous with the middle ear
d) Mastoiditis is commonly related to otitis media

57. The optic nerve: (T/F)
a) Enters the cranium through the ethmoid bone
b) Crosses the midline
c) Can be inflamed in patients with multiple sclerosis
d) Is myelinated

58. The temporomandibular joint: (T/F)
a) Is a synovial joint
b) Is the articulation between the temporal bone and mandibular head
c) Has no capsule
d) Is rarely dislocated in the absence of direct trauma

59. Within the brain: (T/F)
a) The central sulcus separates the frontal lobe from the occipital lobe
b) The lateral sulcus separates the parietal lobe from the temporal lobe
c) The occipital lobe is the smallest lobe
d) The corpus callosum connects the right and left sides of the brain

60. Regarding damaged areas of the brain: (T/F)
a) Damage to Broca's area causes difficulty with speaking
b) Damage to Wernicke's area causes difficulty with limb coordination
c) Damage to the occipital lobe causes hearing problems
d) Posterior cerebral artery occlusion causes visual symptoms

61. The optic nerve: (T/F)
a) Arises within the retina
b) Enters the cranium in the anterior cranial fossa
c) All its fibres cross the midline
d) All the nerve fibres synapse within the lateral geniculate body

62. The internal carotid artery: (T/F)
a) Enters the cranium via the jugular foramen
b) Gives off the opthalmic artery
c) Gives off the occipital artery
d) Gives off the posterior communicating artery

63. The following arteries are components of the circle of Willis: (T/F)
a) Anterior cerebral artery
b) Middle cerebral artery
c) Posterior communicating artery
d) Basilar artery

64. The vagus nerve: (T/F)
a) Arises from the brain stem
b) Leaves the skull through the foramen lacerum
c) Travels in the carotid sheath
d) Passes through the diaphragm through the aortic opening

65. Regarding the spinothalamic tracts: (T/F)
a) They transmit pain and temperature
b) The fibres decussate in the brain stem
c) Are situated anteriorly in the spinal cord
d) Only utilise C fibres to convey nociception

66. The following are correctly paired clinical findings and GCS scores: (T/F)
a) Eyes opening to pain - E2
b) Incomprehensible sounds - V3
c) Abnormal flexion - M3
d) Localises pain - M4

67. Signs of carotid artery dissection include: (T/F)
a) Horner's syndrome
b) Headache
c) Hemiparesis
d) Amaurosis fugax

68. Regarding the external auditory meatus: (T/F)
a) The pinna is a cartilaginous structure
b) The ear canal is approximately 3cm in length
c) Its blood supply is from the facial artery
d) The external surface of the tympanic membrane is supplied solely by the trigeminal nerve

69. Within the eyeball: (T/F)
a) The sclera lies anterior to the cornea
b) The sclera never connects with the cornea
c) The choroid has a pigmented layer
d) The ciliary muscles change the shape of the lens

70. The middle cerebral artery: (T/F)
a) Is the largest branch of the internal carotid artery
b) Supplies the entire motor cortex
c) When occluded, causes a contralateral hemiplegia affecting the face
d) When occluded, causes a sensory loss of the ipsilateral sensory loss affecting the arm

71. The following movements of the jaw are correctly associated with the named muscles: (T/F)
a) Jaw protrusion - medial pterygoid
b) Jaw retraction - temporalis
c) Mouth opening - digastric
d) Mouth closing - lateral pterygoid

72. The sternocleidomastoid muscle: (T/F)
a) Is supplied by the accessory nerve
b) Has the external jugular vein deep to it
c) Divides the neck into anterior and posterior triangles
d) Has platysma superficial to it

73. The internal jugular vein: (T/F)
a) Commences as the continuation of the sagittal sinus
b) Runs in the carotid sheath
c) Contributes to the formation of the brachiocephalic vein
d) Receives the venous drainage of the entire thyroid gland

74. The posterior triangle of the neck: (T/F)
a) Is bounded anteriorly by the sternocleidomastoid
b) Is bounded posteriorly by the trapezius
c) Has the inferior belly of omohyoid as its inferior border
d) Has the insertion of the sternocleidomastoid as its apex

75. Regarding the thyroid gland: (T/F)
a) It has the carotid sheath running anterolaterally to it
b) It has the infrahyoid muscles posterior to it
c) Its isthmus lies in the midline anterior to the 2nd to 4th tracheal rings
d) It is surrounded by a fascial sheath

76. The phrenic nerve: (T/F)
a) Arises from the 3rd to 5th cervical nerves
b) Descends medial to the vagus nerve within the thorax
c) Runs medially to the roots of each lung
d) Passes anteriorly to the scalenus anterior

77. The external jugular vein: (T/F)
a) Runs deep to the sternocleidomastoid
b) Is formed by the union of the posterior auricular and the temporal vein
c) Drains into the subclavian vein
d) Runs deep to platysma

78. Regarding the extrinsic orbital muscles: (T/F)
a) Superior oblique rotates the eye to look upwards and outwards
b) Medial rectus rotates the eye to look inwards
c) Inferior rectus can be damaged in orbital floor fractures
d) Lateral rectus is innervated by the oculomotor nerve

79. Regarding the ventricular system of the brain: (T/F)
a) CSF is produced in all parts of the ventricular system
b) CSF travels between the lateral ventricles and the 3rd ventricle via the foramen of Luschka
c) CSF travels between the 3rd and 4th ventricles via the cerebral aquaduct
d) CSF drains into the venous system via the superior sagittal sinus

80. Orbicularis oris: (T/F)
a) Is supplied by the buccal branch of the facial nerve
b) Arises entirely from the maxilla and mandible
c) Closes the mouth
d) Surrounds the entire mouth

SPINE QUESTIONS

1. The following vertebral groups have the correct number of vertebrae: (T/F)
a) Thoracic - 12
b) Lumbar - 5
c) Sacral - 3
d) Coccygeal - 3

2. Regarding examination findings in spinal injury: (T/F)
a) A patient with grade 2 motor function will be able to lift a limb against gravity
b) An intact bulbocavernosus reflex means that sacral sparing is conclusively present
c) A patient with grade 1 motor function will have visible muscular contractions
d) Lack of spinal tenderness means that the vertebral bodies are intact

3. Each vertebrae contains: (T/F)
a) 4 pedicles
b) 1 spinous process
c) 2 transverse process
d) 2 articular processes

4. Regarding the intervertebral discs: (T/F)
a) The intervertebral discs are thicker in the thoracic region than in the cervical region
b) The anulus fibrosus attaches to the anterior longitudinal ligament only
c) The nucleus pulposus becomes dehydrated with age
d) There are no discs in the sacrum

5. Regarding the spinal ligaments: (T/F)
a) The ligamentum flavum connects the spinous processes of adjacent vertebrae
b) The supraspinous ligament connects the spinous process of one vertebrae to the transverse process of the adjacent vertebrae
c) The interspinous ligament connects the spinous process of one vertebrae to the spinous process of the adjacent vertebrae
d) The ligamentum nuchae is only present in the cervical vertebrae

6. Regarding the atlanto-occipital joints: (T/F)
a) The atlanto-occipital joints are not synovial joints
b) The atlanto-occipital joints have capsules
c) The anterior altlanto-occipital membrane connects the arch of the atlas to the foramen magnum
d) Rotation is possible at the atlanto-occipital joints

7. Anterior cord syndrome: (T/F)
a) Causes a loss of proprioception and light touch
b) Causes complete paralysis below the injury
c) Causes loss of pain below the injury
d) Has an excellent prognosis

8. The following structures are clearly visible on a correctly positioned odontoid peg radiograph: (T/F)
a) Lateral mass of C1
b) Body of C2
c) Dens
d) Spinous process of C1

9. The first cervical vertebrae: (T/F)
a) Has no spinous process
b) Has a vertebral body
c) Has no transverse processes
d) Articulates with the occipital condyles

10. Regarding the atlantoaxial joints: (T/F)
a) The atlantoaxial joints are synovial joints
b) The atlantoaxial joints have capsules
c) There are 2 atlantoaxial joints
d) There is no rotation at the atlantoaxial joints

11. Regarding the layers of the meninges: (T/F)
a) The dura mater surrouding the spine is continuous with the dura of the brain
b) The arachnoid mater is semi-permeable to fluid
c) The sub-arachnoid space lies between the pia and the arachnoid mater
d) The dura does not envelop the spinal nerve roots

12. Brown-Sequard syndrome: (T/F)
a) Is the result of complete spinal cord transection
b) Is more common in penetrating injuries than blunt injuries
c) Causes ipsilateral loss of pain and temperature sensation
d) Causes ipsilateral loss of power and sensation

13. Regarding the ligaments of the atlantoaxial joints: (T/F)
a) The vertical part of the cruciate ligament connects the axis to the foramen magnum
b) The transverse part of the cruciate ligament connects the odontoid process to the atlas
c) The alar ligaments connect the odontoid process to the transverse process of the atlas
d) The apical ligament connects the odontoid process to the foramen magnum

14. The spinal cord: (T/F)
a) In adults, ends at the lower border of the L1 vertebrae
b) Is surrounded by 4 meningeal layers
c) Is continuous with the medulla oblongata
d) Has 4 fissures

15. Regarding the spinal nerves: (T/F)
a) There are 31 pairs of spinal nerves
b) The anterior nerve roots are motor
c) The spinal nerves unite to form the anterior and posterior rami before they pass through the intervertebral foramen
d) The anterior rami only contain sensory fibres

16. During a correctly performed lumbar puncture, the needle passes through the: (T/F)
a) Supraspinous ligament
b) Ligamentum flavum
c) Ligamentum nuchae
d) Erector spinae

17. Viewed from the side, the following descriptions of the spine are correct: (T/F)
a) The cervical spine is posteriorly concave
b) The lumbar spine is posteriorly concave
c) A pregnant woman will have a decreased lumbar posterior concavity
d) An older person will develop an exaggerated posterior thoracic convexity

18. Central cord syndrome: (T/F)
a) Is more common in children than adults
b) The paresis affects the lower limbs more than the upper limbs
c) Characteristically has a fracture visible on plain x-rays
d) Has a variable pattern of sensory deficit

19. The following structures are clearly visible on a lateral cervical spine radiograph: (T/F)
a) Vertebral bodies
b) Spinous processes
c) Transverse processes
d) Facet joints

20. Spinal cord injury without radiographic injury (SCIWORA): (T/F)
a) Can be caused by extradural haematoma
b) Only occurs in children
c) Has a characteristic pattern of neurological deficit
d) Can be caused by ligamentous instability

Answers & explanatory notes

ABDOMEN ANSWERS

1. Internal oblique: (T/F)
a) Inserts into the lower ribs (T-the fibres of internal oblique attach into the lower 6 or 7 ribs)
b) Contributes to rotation of the vertebral column (T)
c) Is innervated by the iliohypogastric nerve (T-as well as the intercostal nerves, internal oblique is innervated by the iliohypogastric nerve and (sometimes) from the ilioinguinal nerve)
d) Originates from the iliac crest (T-as well as the lumbodorsal fascia and the inguinal ligament, the internal oblique originates largely from the iliac crest)

2. Regarding ovarian pathology: (T/F)
a) Pain originating from the ovary can be referred to the medial thigh (T-the ovary is in close relation to the obturator nerve. Pain due to ovarian pathology can therefore be referred to the medial aspect of the thigh, which is supplied by the obturator nerve)
b) Pain originating from the ovary can be referred to the flank and loin (T-the nerve supply to the ovary is from the aortic plexus. These sympathetic fibres cause pain in the T10 and T11 dermatomes)
c) Inguinal lymphadenopathy is not a feature of ovarian pathology (F-the ovaries drain to the para-aortic lymph nodes, but inguinal lymphadenopathy is a known feature of ovarian carcinoma)
d) The ovary can be positioned in the pouch of Douglas (recto-uterine pouch) (T-after pregnancy, the broad ligament becomes lax, allowing the ovary to drop into the recto-uterine pouch. This can be a cause of dyspareunia)

3. Porto-systemic anastomoses can be found: (T/F)
a) At the upper 1/3 of the oesophagus (F-porto-systemic anastomoses are found at the lower 1/3 of the oesophagus

where the oesophageal branches of the left gastric vein (portal circulation) anastomose with the oesophageal veins that drain the middle third of the oesophagus into the azygous veins (systemic circulation). This is the site of oesophageal varices)
b) Halfway down the anal canal (T-the superior rectal veins (portal circulation) which drain the upper half of the anal canal anastomose with the inferior and middle rectal veins (systemic circulation) which drain the lower half of the anal canal. These vessels form the rectal venous plexus, which is the site of haemorrhoid formation)
c) In the paraumbilical veins (T-the para-umbilical veins are the anastomosis of the left branch of the portal vein and the superficial veins of the abdominal wall (systemic circulation). This gives rise to the clinical sign of 'caput medusae', the appearance of dilated veins seen in the periumbilical region of patients with portal hypertension)
d) In the retroperitoneum (T-the right, left and middle colic veins (portal circulation) anastomose with the renal, lumbar and phrenic veins (systemic circulation))

4. Regarding the pelvic ligaments: (T/F)
a) The sacrotuberous membrane runs from the lateral aspect of the sacrum to the iliac crest (F-the sacrotuberous membrane runs from the lateral aspect of the sacrum, the lateral aspect of the coccyx and the iliac spine to the ischial tuberosity)
b) The sacrospinous ligament runs from the lateral part of the sacrum to the spine of the ischium (T-the sacrospinous ligament also arises from the lateral part of the coccyx)
c) The iliolumbar ligament runs from the spinous process of the 5th lumbar vertebra to the iliac crest (F-the iliolumbar ligament runs from the transverse process of the 5th lumbar vertebra to the iliac crest)
d) The sacrococcygeal joint is immobile (F-the

sacrococcygeal joint has a degree of mobility facilitated by the sacrococcygeal and dorsal ligaments)

5. The rectus sheath: (T/F)
a) Is formed by the aponeurosis of the rectus abdominis muscle (F-the rectus sheath is formed by the aponeurosis of the internal and external obliques and the transversus abdominis)
b) Has the linea alba in the midline (T)
c) Has the peritoneum immediately deep to it (F-the transversalis fascia is the immediate layer deep to the sheath. The peritoneum is deep to the transversalis fascia)
d) Has pyramidalis lying superficially to it (F-the pyramidalis is contained within the rectus sheath rather than lying superficial to it)

6. The pancreas: (T/F)
a) Produces glucagon from the beta cells (F-glucagon is produced by the alpha cells of the Islets of Langerhans, insulin is produced by the beta cells)
b) Crosses the midline (T-the body passes across the midline)
c) Lies on the transpyloric plane (T-the body of the pancreas lies on the transpyloric plane at the lower margin of the 1st lower lumbar vertebra)
d) Produces pancreatic lipase from the delta cells of the Islets of Langerhans (F-the production of pancreatic lipase, as well as other digestive enzymes is an exocrine function of the pancreas, taking place in the pancreatic acini. The production of insulin and glucagon is an endocrine function which takes place in the Islets of Langerhans)

7. The inferior epigastric artery: (T/F)
a) Is a branch of the internal iliac artery (F-the inferior

epigastric artery is a branch of the external iliac artery)
b) Runs between the rectus sheath and rectus abdominis (T)
c) Anastomoses with intercostal arteries (T-it anastomoses with the inferior intercostal arteries)
d) Is related to the broad ligament at its origin (F-the round ligament of the uterus, or vas deferens in males, winds around the lateral and posterior aspects of the artery)

8. Regarding the blood supply of the liver: (T/F)
a) The hepatic artery gives off the right and left hepatic arteries after it has entered the liver (F-the hepatic artery gives off the right and left hepatic arteries, which supply the right and left lobes respectively as it enters the porta hepatis, prior to entering the liver parenchyma)
b) The portal vein divides into right and left branches in the porta hepatis, prior to entering the liver (T)
c) The hepatic veins drain directly into the inferior vena cava (T)
d) The portal vein is formed by the union of the inferior mesenteric vein and the splenic vein (F-the portal vein is formed by the union of the superior mesenteric vein and the splenic vein)

9. Regarding the inguinal ligament: (T/F)
a) It runs from the anterior superior iliac spine to the pubic tubercle (T)
b) It is comprised of the inferior border of the internal oblique aponeurosis (F-the inguinal ligament is the lower border of the aponeurosis of the external oblique)
c) It lies above the spermatic cord (F-it lies below the spermatic cord)
d) It becomes continuous with the fascia lata in the thigh (T-the general direction of the inguinal ligament is convex downward toward the thigh, where it is continuous with

the fascia lata)

10. Regarding the male urethra: (T/F)
a) The widest part of the urethra is the membranous urethra (F-the widest part of the urethra is the prostatic urethra)
b) The narrowest part of the urethra is the membranous urethra (F-the membranous urethra is the shortest and least dilatable part of the membranous urethra
c) The external opening of the urethra at the glans is the narrowest part of the urethra (T-this should be considered when carrying out urinary catherisation)
d) The urethra passes through the corpus spongiosum of the penis (T)

11. The floor of the inguinal ligament is comprised of the following: (T/F)
a) The inguinal ligament (T)
b) The lacunar ligament (T)
c) The transversalis fascia (F-the transversalis fascia is part of the posterior wall of the inguinal ligament)
d) The conjoint tendon (F-the conjoint tendon is part of the superior wall of the inguinal ligament-the 'roof')

12. Meckel's diverticulum: (T/F)
a) Arises from the distal jejunum (F-Meckels diverticulum arises from the distal Ileum)
b) Is in close proximity to the iliocaecal valve (T-the 'rule of 2s' -see below, suggests that a Meckels diverticulum will be 2 feet from the ileocaecal valve)
c) Is the remnant of the vitelline duct (T)
d) Has an average length of 10cm (F-the average length is 5 cm, or 2 inches)

Meckel's diverticulum: The 'Rule of 2s'
2% of the population are affected, the location is 2 feet from the ileocaecal valve, the diverticulum is 2 inches in length, 2% of patients are symptomatic, 2 years is the most common age at clinical presentation, 2:1 is the M/F ratio

13. The testicular artery: (T/F)
a) Is a branch of the abdominal aorta (T)
b) Gives a supply to the ureter (T)
c) Passes through the superficial inguinal ring (F-it passes through the deep inguinal ring as part of the spermatic cord)
d) Originates from the supra-renal aorta (F-the spermatic artery is a branch of the infra-renal portion of the aorta)

14. The peritoneum: (T/F)
a) Is a 2 layered structure (T-the visceral and parietal layers make up the peritoneum)
b) Is a non-serous membrane (F-the peritoneum is a serous membrane, it secretes serous fluid)
c) Contains the whole of the small bowel (F-only the first 5 cm of the duodenum is peritoneal, the rest is retroperitoneal)
d) Is a selectively permeable membrane (T-this property is utilised in peritoneal dialysis)

15. The transverse mesocolon: (T/F)
a) Connects the transverse colon to the liver (F-the transverse mesocolon connects the transverse colon to the posterior abdominal wall)
b) Contains the middle colic vessels (T)
c) Is continuous with the lesser omentum (F-it is continuous with the greater omentum)
d) Separates the supracolic and the infracolic components (T)

16. The superficial inguinal ring: (T/F)
a) Is a defect in the aponeurosis of internal oblique (F-it is a defect in the aponeurosis of external oblique)
b) Has the crest of the pubis below it (T)
c) Has the spermatic cord passing through it (T)
d) Has the iliohypogastric nerve passing through it (F-the ilioinguinal nerve passes through the superficial inguinal ring, as does the spermatic cord in males and the round ligament in females)

17. The kidneys: (T/F)
a) Are retroperitoneal (T)
b) Are enclosed in a capsule (T-the fibrous capsule is closely adherent to the outermost surface of the kidney)
c) Have no exterior fascia (F-the renal fascia, known as Gerota's fascia, is a layer of areolar connective tissue which encloses each kidney and the adrenal glands)
d) Move inferiorly by 2 to 2.5 cm during respiration (T)

18. Regarding the infracolic compartment: (T/F)
a) It is divided into the right and left infracolic compartments by the small intestinal mesentery (T-the root of the mesentery of the small intestine divides the infracolic compartment)
b) Receptors within the small bowel mesentery can cause hypotension in the absence of haemorrhage (T-Pacinian corpuscles containing mechanoreceptors can be stimulated by traction and/or tension on the peritoneal folds, causing hypotension)
c) The right infracolic space is larger than the left (F-the left infracolic space is larger than the right)
d) The left ureter crosses the border between the right and left infracolic compartments (F-the ureters are retroperitoneal and hence are not within the infracolic compartment)

19. Contents of the inguinal canal include: (T/F)
a) The spermatic cord (T)
b) The broad ligament (F-the inguinal canal contains the round ligament)
c) The iliohypogastric nerve (F-the inguinal canal contains the ilioinguinal nerve)
d) The aponeurosis of external oblique (F-the aponeurosis of external oblique forms part of the anterior wall of the inguinal canal)

20. Concerning the greater omentum: (T/F)
a) It has a blood supply from a branch of the coeliac trunk (T-the omentum is supplied by the right and left gastroepiploic arteries, both branches of the coeliac trunk)
b) Its content of adipose tissue is not increased in obese people (F-obese people have a greater proportion of adipose tissue within the greater omentum)
c) It contributes to the immune system (T-the greater omentum contains well organised, macrophage-rich areas which contribute to the abdominal immune system)
d) It is attached to the lesser curve of the stomach (F -the greater omentum descends from the greater curve of the stomach and subsequently ascends towards the transverse colon. It crosses the duodenum and gives attachment to the gastrosplenic ligament)

21. Regarding renal pathology: (T/F)
a) A perirenal abscess involves spread of pus into the retroperitoneal space (F-the extent of a perirenal abscess is limited by the renal fascia. Occasionally the fascia can rupture and pus can spread into the pararenal fat and beyond)
b) 'Renal' pain is felt in the T12 dermatome (T-the kidney has afferent nerve fibres which transmit to the renal plexus and then to the spinal cord at the level of T12 via

the least splanchnic nerve and the sympathetic trunk. The pain is referred along the distribution of the subcostal nerve (from T12) towards the flank)
c) Ureteric colic causes pain to be felt in the T11 and T12 dermatomes only (F-the spasms caused by ureteric colic cause afferent transmission to the spinal segments T11 to L2, hence the pain being felt from the flank down to the loin and groin)
d) Flank pain is not a feature of renal infarction (F-back and flank pain are common in renal infarction, although it can be asymptomatic. Renal infarction is often initially misdiagnosed as renal colic or ascending urinary tract infection)

22. Regarding the oesophagus: (T/F)
a) The cardiac orifice is at the level of the 12th thoracic vertebra (F-the cardiac orifice is at the level of the 10th thoracic vertebra, to the left of the midline)
b) It is supplied by the vagus nerve (T-the supply to the oesophagus is via the vagus nerve and sympathetic fibres from the coeliac plexus)
c) The posterior aspect of the abdominal oesophagus is covered with peritoneum (F-only its front and left aspects are covered by peritoneum)
d) It has a blood supply derived from the abdominal aorta (T-the oesophagus derives its blood supply from the inferior thyroid branch of the thyrocervical trunk, from the descending thoracic aorta, from the left gastric branch of the coeliac artery and from the left inferior phrenic branch of the abdominal aorta)

23. The following are contents of the spermatic cord: (T/F)
a) Testicular artery (T)
b) Genitofemoral nerve (T-the genital branch of the genitofemoral nerve lies within the spermatic cord)
c) Ilioinguinal nerve (F)

d) Pampiniform plexus (T)

The contents of the spermatic cord are:
Arteries-testicular artery, the artery of the vas deferens and the cremasteric artery
Veins-testicular veins (pampiniform plexus)
Nerves-genital branch of the genitofemoral nerve, testicular nerves
Vas deferens
Lymphatic vessels
Remnants of the processus vaginalis

24. Regarding the liver: (T/F)
a) The liver is the largest organ in the human body (T)
b) The right and left lobes are separated by the ligamentum teres (F-the attachment of the peritoneum of the falciform ligament separates the right and left lobes)
c) The left lobe is larger than the right lobe (F-the right lobe is the larger of the two lobes)
d) It is completely covered by peritoneum (F-the liver is completely surrounded by a fibrous capsule, but its peritoneal covering is incomplete)

25. Regarding the stomach: (T/F)
a) The fundus is located inferiorly to the cardiac orifice (F-the fundus, especially its uppermost surface, sits superior to the cardiac orifice)
b) The lesser curvature gives attachment to the hepatogastric ligament (T)
c) The pyloric antrum secretes somatostatin and insulin (F-the pyloric antrum secretes somatostatin and gastrin)
d) The pyloric sphincter has a layer of striated muscle (F-the pyloric sphincter is a ring of smooth muscle that facilitates the transmission of food to the duodenum)

26. External oblique: (T/F)
a) Originates from the lower eight ribs (T)
b) Forms the superior wall (roof) of the inguinal canal (F-external oblique contributes to the anterior wall of the inguinal canal. The roof of the inguinal canal is formed by the internal oblique and transversus abdominis)
c) Forms the linea alba in the midline (T-the linea alba is formed from the aponeurosis of external oblique on either side of the midline)
d) Inserts into the iliac crest (T-as well as the iliac crest, the external oblique also inserts into the inguinal ligament and, via its aponeurosis, the linea alba)

27. The nerve supply of the stomach: (T/F)
a) Is derived from the vagus nerve (T)
b) Has separate branches to the anterior and posterior aspects (T)
c) Is derived from the coeliac plexus (T)
d) Is contained within the submucosa (F-see below)

The nerves supplying the stomach are derived from the vagus, in the form of right and left branches. The right branch is distributed to the posterior surface and the left to the anterior surface. A number of branches from the coeliac plexus of the sympathetic system also supply the stomach. Nerve plexuses are found in the submucosal layer coat and between the layers of the muscular coat as in the intestine. From these plexuses, fibres are distributed to the muscular tissue and the mucous membrane

28. The porta hepatis: (T/F)
a) Is on the posterior surface of the liver (T-the porta hepatis is on the posteroinferior aspect of the liver)
b) Has no attachment to the omentum (F-the superior part of the lesser omentum has an attachment to the porta hepatis)

c) Contains the portal vein (T)
d) Contains the hepatic ducts (T)

The contents of the porta hepatis are the right and left hepatic ducts, the portal vein and the hepatic artery, which divides into its right and left branches as it enters the porta hepatis. The porta hepatis also transmits various lymphatics and nerves

29. Scarpa's fascia: (T/F)
a) Is deep to the external oblique muscle (F-Scarpa's fascia is superficial to the external oblique)
b) Is adherent to the linea alba (T-Scarpa's fascia is loosely connected to the aponeurosis of the external oblique, but in the midline it is more intimately adherent to the linea alba)
c) Descends to the scrotum (T-Scarpa's fascia blends with the deep fascia of the thigh (fascia lata) a little below the inguinal ligament. It then continues over the penis and spermatic cord to the scrotum, where it helps to form the dartos fascia)
d) Is thicker than the superficial fascia (F-Scarpa's fascia is is thinner and more membranous in character than the superficial fascia)

30. Regarding the duodenum: (T/F)
a) It has a blood supply derived from the superior mesenteric artery (T-the inferior pancreaticoduodenal branch of the superior mesenteric supplies the duodenum)
b) It has a blood supply derived from the hepatic artery (T-the superior pancreaticoduodenal artery supplies the duodenum and pancreas. It is a branch of the gastroduodenal artery which most commonly arises from the common hepatic artery)

c) Its venous drainage is to the inferior mesenteric vein (F-the duodenum drains via the pancreaticoduodenal veins to the portal vein and the superior mesenteric vein)
d) The head of the pancreas lies on the transpyloric plane (F-the neck and body of the pancreas lies on the transpyloric plane, the head lies inferior to it)

31. The vermiform appendix: (T/F)
a) Arises from the base of the caecum (T)
b) Derives its blood supply from the inferior mesenteric artery (F-the appendix is supplied by the appendicular artery, a branch of the ileocolic artery, which is a branch of the superior mesenteric artery)
c) Is always intraperitoneal (F-the tip of the appendix has a variable length and position. The base of the appendix is classically located 2 cm below the ileocaecal valve. However the tip can lie behind the caecum, within the pelvis, or occasionally outside of the peritoneum. These variations in location explain the highly variable presentation of appendicitis)
d) Does not have a muscular layer (F-the appendix has longitudinal and circular muscle layers)

32. The ascending colon: (T/F)
a) Is retroperitoneal (T)
b) Passes medially to the gallbladder below the liver (F-the ascending colon ascends towards the liver where it turns acutely at the hepatic flexure. It leaves an impression on the inferior surface of the liver-the colic impression, which lies lateral to the gallbladder)
c) Is supplied by a branch of the superior mesenteric artery (T-the right colic artery supplies the ascending colon. It is a branch of the superior mesenteric artery)
d) Has the inferolateral aspect of the right kidney posterior to it as it ascends to the hepatic flexure (T)

33. The duodenum: (T/F)
a) Is the longest part of the small intestine (F-the duodenum is the shortest part of the small intestine)
b) Is entirely covered by mesentery (F)
c) Has the head of the pancreas posterior and inferior to its first part (T)
d) Has the aorta posterior to its third part (T)

34. Regarding the inferior vena cava: (T/F)
a) It has a variable number of anterior visceral tributaries (T-the inferior vena cava receives the hepatic veins anteriorly. There can be a variation in the number of hepatic veins a patient has. They are arranged in two groups, upper and lower. There are normally 3 veins in the upper group and a variable number in the lower group)
b) It receives 2 suprarenal veins (F-the left suprarenal vein drains into the left renal vein, then into the inferior vena cava. The right renal vein drains directly into the inferior vena cava)
c) It receives the renal veins at the level of the L1 vertebra (T)
d) It receives the left testicular vein directly (F-the left testicular vein drains into the left renal vein. The right testicular vein drains directly into the inferior vena cava)

35. The sigmoid colon: (T/F)
a) Becomes continuous with the rectum anterior to the 3rd sacral vertebra (T)
b) Is supplied by branches of the iliac arteries (F-the sigmoid colon is supplied by sigmoid branches of the inferior mesenteric artery)
c) Is completely covered by peritoneum (T)
d) Receives parasympathetic supply directly from the vagus nerve (F-the sympathetic and parasympathetic supply is via the inferior hypogastric plexuses (C2 to C4))

36. Regarding the abdominal aorta: (T/F)
a) It gives off 4 lateral visceral branches (F-the abdominal aorta gives off 3 lateral visceral branches-the suprarenal, the renal and the testicular/ovarian arteries)
b) It gives off 5 lateral abdominal branches (T-these are the inferior phrenic artery and the 4 lumbar arteries)
c) It has 2 terminal branches (F-there are 3 terminal branches-the median sacral artery and the right and left common iliac arteries)
d) It has 3 anterior visceral branches (T-these are the superior and inferior mesenteric arteries and the coeliac artery)

37. The following are part of the direct arterial supply to the stomach: (T/F)
a) Left gastric artery (T)
b) Hepatic artery (F-see below)
c) Splenic artery (F-see below)
d) Right gastroepiploic artery (T)

The lesser curvature of the stomach *is supplied by the right gastric artery (from the common hepatic artery) inferiorly, and the left gastric artery (from the coeliac artery) superiorly. The left gastric artery also supplies the cardia.*
The greater curvature is supplied by the right gastroepiploic (from the gastroduodenal artery) inferiorly and the left gastroepiploic artery (from the splenic artery) superiorly. The fundus and the upper portion of the greater curvature are supplied by the short gastric artery (from the splenic artery)

38. Regarding the biliary ducts: (T/F)
a) The common hepatic duct is formed by union of the right and left hepatic ducts only (T-the common hepatic duct is formed by union of the right and left hepatic ducts. The common bile duct is formed by the union of the common hepatic duct and the cystic duct from the

gallbladder)
b) The common bile duct runs through the greater omentum (F-the common bile duct runs between the 2 layers of the lesser omentum, close to the portal vein and the hepatic artery)
c) The common bile duct forms the ampulla of Vater when it is joined by the pancreatic duct (T-the union of the common bile duct and the pancreatic duct is known as the ampulla of Vater. The ampulla opens into the duodenum at the major duodenal papilla)
d) The ampulla of Vater is surrounded by a circular layer of smooth muscle (T-the sphincter of Oddi surrounds the ampulla of Vater and the terminal portions of the common bile duct and the pancreatic duct)

39. The transverse colon: (T/F)
a) Is the least mobile part of the colon (F-the transverse colon is the most mobile part of the colon)
b) Is connected to the pancreas and the posterior abdominal wall by the transverse mesocolon (T)
c) Is supplied by the middle colic artery (T)
d) Runs anterior to the greater curvature of the stomach (F-the transverse colon runs inferior to the greater curvature of the stomach)

40. Regarding the liver: (T/F)
a) The left lobe is divided into the caudate lobe and the quadrate lobe (F-the right lobe is divided into the caudate lobe and the quadrate lobe)
b) The gallbladder is the only structure that forms the division between the caudate and quadrate lobes (F-the right lobe is subdivided into the caudate and quadrate lobes by the gallbladder, the fissure for the ligamentum teres, the fissure for the ligamentum venosum and the inferior vena cava)
c) The fissure containing the ligamentum teres lies

between the left lobe and the quadrate lobe (T-the ligamentum teres is the fibrous remnant of the umbilical vein)
d) The fissure for the ligamentum venosum lies between the left lobe and the caudate lobe (T-the ligamentum venosum is the fibrous remnant of the ductus venosus)

41. The descending colon: (T/F)
a) Descends between psoas major and quadratus lumborum (T)
b) Lies lateral to the right kidney (T)
c) Is supplied by branches of the superior mesenteric artery (F-the descending colon is supplied by the left colic artery and the sigmoid artery, both are branches of the inferior mesenteric artery)
d) Has its venous drainage directly into the inferior vena cava (F-the venous drainage is into the inferior mesenteric vein)

42. The jejunum: (T/F)
a) Does not have a mesenteric attachment (F-the jejunum is suspended by a mesentery)
b) Has a wider lumen than the ileum (T)
c) Derives its blood supply from the superior mesenteric artery (T-the jejunal arteries are branches of the superior mesenteric artery)
d) Can be a cause of referred pain in the T9/T10 dermatomes (T)

43. Regarding the liver: (T/F)
a) The coronary ligament attaches the liver to the greater omentum (F-the coronary ligament attaches the liver to the diaphragm)
b) The coronary ligament is comprised of 2 reflected layers of visceral peritoneum (T)

c) The bare area of the liver is the area which has no peritoneal covering (T-this area is triangular in shape and is attached to the diaphragm by areolar connective tissue)
d) The bare area is not covered by the fibrous liver capsule (F-the liver capsule completely surrounds the liver)

44. Regarding the lumbar plexus: (T/F)
a) It is formed by the 1st to 5th lumbar nerves (F-the lumbar plexus is formed from the 1st to 4th lumbar nerves)
b) It is situated within the psoas muscle (T)
c) The femoral nerve arises from the lumbar plexus (T-the femoral nerve arises from the first 3 lumbar nerves)
d) The nerve to the quadratus femoris arises from the lumbar plexus (F-the nerve to the quadratus femoris arises from the sacral plexus)

45. Regarding the triangular ligaments: (T/F)
a) The right triangular ligament is formed by the layers of the coronary ligament (T)
b) The right triangular ligament connects the liver to the diaphragm (T-the right triangular ligament connects the posterior aspect of the right lobe to the diaphragm)
c) The left triangular ligament is continuous with the coronary ligament (F-the left triangular ligament is continuous with the falciform ligament)
d) The left triangular ligament connects the liver to the diaphragm (T-the left triangular ligament connects the posterior surface of the left lobe to the diaphragm)

46. The gallbladder: (T/F)
a) Has an arterial blood supply from the left hepatic artery (F-the gallbladder is supplied by the cystic artery, a branch of the right hepatic artery)
b) Contracts in response to a hormone produced in the duodenum (T-cholecystokinin is produced in the mucous

membrane of the duodenum as a response to the presence of food after gastric emptying)
c) Is continuous with the cystic duct (T-the neck of the gallbladder is continuous with the cystic duct)
d) Is separated from the liver by a layer of peritoneum (F-there is no peritoneum between the gallbladder and the liver)

47. Regarding the portal vein: (T/F)
a) It is formed by the union of the superior mesenteric vein and the splenic vein (T)
b) It drains blood from the spleen (T)
c) It drains blood from the bile ducts (T)
d) It drains blood from the pancreas (T)

48. The testicles: (T/F)
a) Have their lymphatic drainage to the para-aortic nodes (T)
b) Have bilateral venous drainage directly to the inferior vena cava (F-the right testicular vein generally joins the inferior vena cava, but the left testicular vein joins the left renal vein. This renders it more susceptible to varicocele due to the higher pressures that can develop between the left testicle and the left kidney)
c) Descend in utero through the inguinal canal (T)
d) Can survive for 24 hours following testicular torsion (F-surgery to correct testicular torsion must take place within 12 hours if the testicle(s) are to survive. The quicker surgery is carried out, the more likely the chance of success)

49. The pancreas: (T/F)
a) Derives its blood supply from the splenic artery (T-the pancreas is also supplied by the superior and inferior pancreaticoduodenal arteries, branches of the gastroduodenal and superior mesenteric arteries

respectively)
b) Has its venous drainage directly into the portal vein (T)
c) Is associated with referred pain to the T6 to T10 dermatomes (T-the pancreas sends visceral nociceptive afferents to these spinal segments)
d) Is situated within the peritoneum (F-the pancreas is retroperitoneal)

50. The spleen: (T/F)
a) Is not surrounded by peritoneum (F-the spleen is surrounded by peritoneum, which forms the gastrosplenic and splenorenal ligaments)
b) Is retroperitoneal (F-the spleen is intraperitoneal)
c) Is supplied by a branch of the superior mesenteric artery (F-the spleen is supplied by the splenic artery, which is a branch of the coeliac artery)
d) Has its venous drainage into the portal system (T-the splenic vein unites with the superior mesenteric vein to form the portal vein)

51. The abdominal aorta: (T/F)
a) Enters the abdomen through the diaphragm at the level of the T10 vertebra (F-the aorta enters the abdomen through the diaphragm at the level of the T12 vertebra)
b) Divides into the common iliac arteries at the level of the 4th lumbar vertebra (T)
c) Gives off the renal artery as its first branch (F-the inferior phrenic artery, the coeliac artery, the superior mesenteric artery and the suprarenal artery are given off above the renal arteries)
d) Descends anterior to the lumbar vertebral bodies (T)

52. Regarding the surface of the liver: (T/F)
a) The groove for the inferior vena cava lies between the right and left lobes (F-the groove for the inferior vena cava lies between the right lobe and the caudate lobe)

b) The fossa containing the gallbladder lies between the right lobe and the caudate lobe (T)
c) The area between the gallbladder and the liver is covered with peritoneum (F-there is no peritoneum between the gallbladder and the liver)
d) The hepatic veins join the inferior vena cava adjacent to the junction of the right lobe and the caudate lobe (T)

53. The inferior vena cava: (T/F)
a) Is formed by the union of the iliac and femoral veins (F-the inferior vena cava is formed by the union of the right and left common iliac veins. The median sacral vein also contributes to the origin of the inferior vena cava)
b) Is formed at the level of the L4 vertebra (F-the vena cava is formed at the level of the L5 vertebra)
c) Ascends on the left side of the vertebral column (F-the inferior vena cava ascends to the right of the vertebral column)
d) Enters the diaphragm at the level of the T8 vertebra (T)

54. Regarding gallbladder pathology: (T/F)
a) Gallstones are frequently asymptomatic (T-painful episodes are caused by spasm of the smooth muscle layers of the gallbladder, or by inflammation of the gallbladder. However, people with gallstones are asymptomatic most of the time)
b) Shoulder tip pain indicates irritation of the sub-diaphragmatic peritoneum (T-irritation of the parietal peritoneum in the sub-diaphragmatic area can cause shoulder tip pain, due to involvement of the phrenic nerve (C3 to C5))
c) Biliary colic is always related to the presence of gallstone (F-acalculous biliary colic can occur due to functional disorders of the biliary tree and can occur after cholecystectomy)
d) Cholangitis is inflammation of the gallbladder

(F-cholangitis is inflammation of the biliary tree, cholecystitis is inflammation of the gallbladder)

55. Regarding the kidneys: (T/F)
a) They have no external fat (F-the kidney has both perirenal and pararenal fat layers. The perirenal fat covers the fibrous capsule and the pararenal fat layer covers the renal fascia)
b) The lymphatic drainage of the kidneys is into the para-aortic nodes (T)
c) The left kidney is lower than the right (F-the right kidney is lower than the left due to its position under the right lobe of the liver)
d) They are palpable in normal, healthy individuals (F-the kidney is only palpable when it is enlarged or misplaced)

56. Regarding the bladder: (T/F)
a) The apex points superiorly (F-the apex points anteriorly)
b) The base faces inferiorly (F-the base faces posteriorly)
c) The neck of the bladder points inferiorly (T)
d) The superior surface is covered with peritoneum (T)

57. The following structures can be palpated on a rectal examination in a healthy individual: (T/F)
a) The rectovesical pouch (T)
b) The prostate gland (T)
c) The ovary (F-the ovaries can be palpated by bimanual palpation as part of a vaginal examination. Expanding ovarian masses may be felt on a rectal examination)
d) The cervix (T)

58. Regarding the prostate gland: (T/F)
a) It is not surrounded by a capsule (F-the prostate is enclosed in a fibrous capsule which lies within a fibrous sheath of pelvic fascia)

b) The base of the prostate is adjacent to the femoral neck (T)
c) It is a lobular structure (T)
d) It has its lymphatic drainage to the internal iliac nodes (T)

59. The supracolic compartment contains: (T/F)
a) Stomach (T)
b) Liver (T)
c) Kidneys (F-the kidneys are retroperitoneal, neither supracolic nor infracolic)
d) Spleen (T)

60. The ovaries: (T/F)
a) Are attached to the broad ligament (T-the mesovarium attaches the ovary to the broad ligament)
b) Receive their blood supply via the round ligament (F-the blood and nerve supplies to the ovaries are contained within the suspensory ligament)
c) Receive their blood supply from a direct branch of the abdominal aorta (T-the ovarian artery is a branch of the aorta)
d) Drain directly into the inferior vena cava bilaterally (F-the right ovarian vein drains directly into the inferior vena cava, the left ovarian vein drains into the left renal vein)

61. Regarding the sacral plexus: (T/F)
a) It is formed by the 4th and 5th lumbar and 1st to 4th sacral nerves (T-the anterior rami of these nerves form the sacral plexus)
b) The sciatic nerve arises from the sacral plexus (T-the sciatic nerve is derived from the L4, L5, S1 to S3 nerves)
c) The pudendal nerve is derived from the L4 and L5 nerves (F-the pudendal nerve is derived from the S2 to S4 nerves)

d) The sciatic nerve exits the pelvis via the obturator foramen (F-the sciatic nerve leaves the pelvis through the greater sciatic foramen)

62. The bladder: (T/F)
a) In adults, is pyramidal in shape when empty (T)
b) Becomes circular in shape as it fills (F-the bladder becomes ovoid in shape as it fills)
c) In children, drops down into the pelvis as it fills (T)
d) In adults, displaces the rectum to expand posteriorly as it fills (F-the bladder expands into the abdominal cavity as it fills)

63. Regarding prostate cancer: (T/F)
a) It is an adenocarcinoma (T-prostate cancer occurs when the glandular tissue of the prostate undergoes neoplastic change)
b) Tumour staging involves the number of prostate lobes involved (T)
c) It can spread locally into the rectum (T)
d) It rarely metastases to bone (F-bone metastases are common in patients with prostate cancer)

64. The infracolic compartment contains: (T/F)
a) Small bowel (T)
b) Descending colon (T)
c) Bladder (F-the bladder is retroperitoneal)
d) Ascending colon (T)

65. Regarding the spleen: (T/F)
a) It is essential for life (F-some people are born without a spleen (congenital asplenia), although this is rare. It is occasionally necessary to remove the spleen due to haemorrhage following trauma or to halt the function of the spleen (e.g. idiopathic thrombocytopenic purpura, spherocytosis. Sickle cell disease can cause

autosplenectomy due to hypoxia and splenic infarction, this causes a shrunken and non-functioning spleen)
b) It lies under the 7th to 9th ribs (F-the spleen lies under the lower ribs, classically between the 9th and 11th ribs)
c) It is visible on FAST ultrasound (T-part of the spleen is visible on a FAST scan. More importantly, the appearance of free fluid in the splenorenal angle is an indicator of intraperitoneal haemorrhage)
d) It has a notched posterior border (F-the spleen has a notched anterior border)

THORAX ANSWERS

1. Regarding the dermatomes of the anterior thoracic wall: (T/F)
a) The nipples are within the T4 dermatome (T)
b) The nipples are within the T6 dermatome (F-the nipples are within the T4 dermatome)
c) The umbilicus lies at the T12 dermatome (F-the umbilicus lies at the level of the T10 dermatome)
d) The umbilicus lies at the level of the T10 dermatome (T)

2. Regarding the intercostal muscles: (T/F)
a) There are 12 sets (right and left) of external intercostal muscles (F-there are 11 pairs of external intercostals, extending from the tubercles of the ribs behind, to the cartilages of the ribs in front. They end in thin membranes, the anterior intercostal membranes, which continue forward to the sternum. They are thicker than the internal intercostal muscles and their fibres are directed obliquely downward and laterally on the posterior surface of the thorax, and downward, forward, and medially on the anterior thorax)
b) There are 11 sets of internal intercostal muscles (T-they commence anteriorly at the sternum and extend backward as far as the angles of the ribs. They then continue to the vertebral column via the posterior intercostal membranes. Their fibres are directed obliquely, but pass in a direction opposite to those of the external intercostal muscles)
c) The innermost intercostal muscles contain the intercostal neurovascular bundle (F-the innermost intercostal muscles are deep to the plane that contains the intercostal nerves and vessels)
d) The transversus thoracus muscle arises from the sternum (T-transversus thoracus arises from the lower third of the posterior surface of the sternal body and from

the posterior surface of the xiphisternum. It also arises from the sternal ends of the costal cartilages of the lower 3 or 4 ribs)

3. Regarding the diaphragm: (T/F)
a) The opening for the inferior vena cava is at the level of T10 (F-the caval opening is at the level of T8)
b) The opening for the oesophagus is at the level of T10 (T-this opening also transmits the anterior and posterior vagal trunks, and some of the oesophageal arteries)
c) It is solely innervated by the phrenic nerve (F-peripheral parts of the diaphragm receive their sensory supply from the lower intercostal nerves)
d) A hiatus hernia involves the abdominal oesophagus rising through the oesophageal opening (T-a hiatus hernia involves the abdominal oesophagus and/or fundus of the stomach rising through the oesophageal opening)

4. Regarding the diaphragm: (T/F)
a) Paralysis at the level of C4 will have no effect on diaphragmatic function (F-the main innervation of the diaphragm is by the 3rd, 4th and 5th cervical nerves. Injury to these nerve will affect diaphragmatic function, resulting in respiratory compromise)
b) The opening for the aorta is at the level of T10 (F-the opening for the aorta is at the level of T12. It also transmits the azygos vein and the thoracic duct, although occasionally the azygos vein is transmitted through the right crus of the diaphragm)
c) Congenital hernias of the diaphragm are mostly left sided (T-approximately 85% of Bochdalek hernias, which are the most common congenital diaphragmatic hernia, occur on the left side)
d) The diaphragm relaxes during inhalation (F-during inhalation, the diaphragm contracts, enlarging the thoracic cavity)

5. During a 'clamshell' thoracotomy: (T/F)
a) The internal mammary arteries are not at risk of being damaged (F-dividing the sternum, which is a component of the clamshell thoracotomy, will divide the inferior mammary arteries on both sides)
b) A Gigli saw is used to cut through the ribs (F-a Gigli saw is used to split the sternum. This can also be accomplished by using trauma shears or heavy surgical scissors)
c) The superior part of the mediastinum is easily reached (F-the superior mediastinum is difficult to reach in a clamshell thoracotomy; the sternum must be split to reach this area if necessary)
d) The chest cannot always be surgically closed following a clamshell thoracotomy (T-occasionally attempts to close the chest will result in cardiac arrest as the heart has become so oedematous it does not tolerate the compression)

6. The thoracic inlet: (T/F)
a) Has the 1st thoracic vertebrae posteriorly (T)
b) Has the costal cartilage of the first rib and the superior border of the manubrium anteriorly (T)
c) Transmits the trachea (T)
d) Transmits the phrenic nerve (T)

The thoracic inlet also transmits the innominate vessels, the left common carotid, left subclavian and internal mammary arteries and the costocervical trunks, the vagus, cardiac, phrenic, and sympathetic nerves, the greater parts of the anterior divisions of the first thoracic nerves, and the left recurrent laryngeal nerve

7. The trachea: (T/F)
a) Commences at the level of the 6th cervical vertebrae (T)
b) Has the recurrent laryngeal nerves posterior to it (F-the

recurrent laryngeal nerves run anterolaterally to the trachea)
c) Is reinforced with cartilaginous rings posteriorly and laterally (F-the trachea is reinforced with cartilaginous walls anteriorly and laterally)
d) Lies in the superior mediastinum in the thorax (T)

8. The thymus: (T/F)
a) Has the 5th costal cartilage as its lower border (F-the 4th costal cartilage is the lower border of the thymus)
b) Extends upwards to the lower border of the thyroid (T)
c) Is at its largest during childhood (T-the thymus reaches maximum weight around puberty and then shrinks during adult life)
d) Normally consists of a heterogenous mass (F-it characteristically consists of 2 lobes. However, there is some variation in the appearance of the thymus. It can have more than 2 lobes or can sometimes consist of 1 single mass)

9. Regarding the heart valves: (T/F)
a) The mitral valve has 3 leaflets (F-the mitral valve is bicuspid i.e. has 2 leaflets)
b) The closing of the mitral valve and the tricuspid valve constitutes the first heart sound (T)
c) The aortic valve has 2 leaflets (F)
d) The pulmonary valve has 2 leaflets (F-the pulmonary and aortic valves are both tricuspid. Congenitally bicuspid aortic valves are seen in approximately 1% of the population and also in conditions such as Turner's disease)

10. Regarding the pericardium: (T/F)
a) The serous pericardium has 2 layers (T-the serous pericardium is a closed sac which lines the fibrous pericardium and is invaginated by the heart. It consists of

a visceral and a parietal portion. The visceral portion, otherwise known as the epicardium, covers the heart and the great vessels. The parietal portion is continuous with the fibrous pericardium)
b) The phrenic nerve runs over its surface (T-the phrenic nerve descends between the pericardium and pleura)
c) It is supplied by a branch of the external mammary artery (F-it is supplied by the musculophrenic and pericardiacophrenic arteries, both branches of the internal mammary artery)
d) It has a potential space between the fibrous and serous layers (T-this contains a layer of pericardial fluid which lubricates the pericardium. If fluid accumulates in this layer (e.g. blood or inflammatory exudate) a pericardial effusion will form, which can compromise cardiac function)

11. Regarding the great vessels: (T/F)
a) The aorta gives off the right and left coronary arteries as it leaves the left ventricle (T)
b) The superior vena cava is separated from the right atrium by a valve (F-there is no valve separating the superior vena cava from the right atrium. This allows right ventricular contractions to be visualised as the jugular venous waveform)
c) The pulmonary artery is the only artery in humans to carry de-oxygenated blood (F-the umbilical arteries carry de-oxygenated blood from the foetus to the placenta)
d) The inferior vena cava is retroperitoneal (T-the aorta is also retroperitoneal)

12. The oesophagus: (T/F)
a) Begins at the level of the C6 vertebrae (T)
b) Ends at the level of the T12 vertebrae (F-the oesophagus ends at the level of the T10 vertebrae)
c) Passes posterior to the left main bronchus (T)

d) Enters the abdomen through the diaphragm at the level of the T10 vertebra (T)

13. The oesophagus has specific areas of constriction. These are located: (T/F)
a) Where it is crossed by the thyroid gland (F)
b) Behind the cricoid cartilage (T)
c) Where its anterior surface is crossed by the aortic arch (T)
d) Where it pierces the diaphragm (T)

14. Regarding the lungs: (T/F)
a) The left lung has 3 lobes (F-the left lung has 2 lobes)
b) The right lung has 3 lobes (T)
c) The horizontal fissure lies anteriorly at the level of the 4th costal cartilage (T)
d) The oblique fissure lies anteriorly at the level of the 4th costal cartilage (F-the oblique fissure lies at the level of the sixth costal cartilage)

15. Regarding thoracic injuries: (T/F)
a) A flail chest is defined as a single rib, fractured in 2 places (F-flail chest is defined as 2 adjacent ribs, each fractured in 2 places)
b) Pulmonary contusion is rare when a flail chest is present (F-pulmonary contusions are almost always present when a flail chest is present. It is this pathology which leads to the morbidity and mortality associated with flail chest)
c) Rupture of the right diaphragm is more common than rupture of the left (F-left sided diaphragmatic ruptures account for approximately 75% of these injuries)
d) Sternal fracture may be associated with myocardial contusion (T)

16. The azygos vein: (T/F)
a) Has the pericardial veins draining into it (T)
b) Is the continuation of the left ascending lumbar vein (F-the azygos vein is formed from the union of the right ascending lumbar vein and the right subcostal veins. The hemiazygos vein is formed from the left ascending lumbar vein, although it can arise from the left renal vein)
c) Runs up the right side of the thoracic vertebral column (T)
d) Enters the diaphragm at the level of T10 (F-the azygos vein enters the diaphragm at the level of T12, along with the aorta)

17. Regarding the ribs: (T/F)
a) The upper 6 ribs are attached directly to the sternum (F-the upper 7 ribs are the 'true ribs' i.e. they are attached directly to the sternum)
b) All the ribs are attached to the thoracic vertebrae (T)
c) The lowest 2 ribs are 'floating ribs' (T-the 11th and 12th ribs do not have any anterior connection to the sternum)
d) The 1st rib articulates with the body of the sternum (F-the first rib articulates with the manubrium)

18. Regarding the pleura: (T/F)
a) It has 2 layers (T-the visceral and parietal pleura make up the pleura)
b) The pleural cavity contains no fluid in normal, healthy individuals (F-the pleural cavity always contains a small amount of pleural fluid)
c) The visceral pleura is highly sensitive to pain (F-the parietal pleura is innervated by the phrenic and intercostal nerves and is very sensitive to pain. The visceral pleura is not sensitive to pain)
d) Mesothelioma affects the pleura rather than the lung parenchyma (T)

19. The sinoatrial node: (T/F)
a) Is receptive to sympathetic innervation only (F-the parasympathetic nervous system has a notable effect on the sinoatrial node)
b) Normally has an arterial supply arising from the right coronary artery (T-the supply can less commonly be from the circumflex branch of the left coronary artery)
c) Lies near the entrance of the superior vena cava to the heart (T)
d) Normally has a pacemaker action setting the heart rate at 60 to 100 beats per minute (T)

20. Regarding heart sounds: (T/F)
a) The 1st heart sound is related to the closure of the aortic and pulmonary valves (F-the 1st heart sound corresponds to the closure of the atrioventricular valves)
b) The 2nd heart sound is related to the closure of the aortic and pulmonary valves (T)
c) A split 2nd heart sound can occur in healthy individuals (T-if heard during inspiration, a split S2 is often physiological. If heard outside of inspiration, it can be as a result of aortic stenosis, hypertrophic cardiomyopathy and septal defects)
d) A grade 6 heart murmur requires a stethoscope to hear it (F-a grade 6 murmur is audible without a stethoscope)

UPPER LIMB ANSWERS

1. Regarding shoulder dislocations: (T/F)
a) Luxio erectae is a type of posterior shoulder dislocation (F-luxio erectae is a description of inferior dislocation of the shoulder)
b) Posterior shoulder dislocation is associated with epileptic seizures (T)
c) Anterior shoulder dislocation is associated with permanent axillary nerve injury (F-axillary nerve damage is normally transient when it occurs following shoulder dislocation)
d) Posterior shoulder dislocation rarely has a delay in diagnosis. (F-posterior shoulder dislocation is notorious for its tendency towards delayed diagnosis, especially in the elderly and obtunded trauma patients)

2. The origins of Pectoralis major include: (T/F)
a) The posterior surface of the sternal half of the clavicle (F-the anterior surface of the clavicle is one of the origins of pectoralis major)
b) The anterior surface of the sternum (T)
c) The aponeurosis of the external oblique muscle (T)
d) The cartilages of the 'true ribs' (T)

3. The ulnar nerve: (T/F)
a) Arises from the medial cord of the brachial plexus (T-the ulnar nerve originates from the C8 to T1 nerve root)
b) Supplies the 1st and 2nd lumbrical muscles (F-it supplies the 3rd and 4th lumbricals. The median nerve supplies the 1st and 2nd lumbricals)
c) Innervates all the interossei muscles (T-the dorsal and palmar interossei are supplied by the deep branch of the ulnar nerve)
d) Is involved in Erb's palsy (F-Erb's palsy is caused by the excessive sideways movement of an infants neck during

labour, especially in difficult labour. Klumpke's paralysis involves C8 and T1 and can also be injured during difficult labour, but results from traction on the abducted arm, such as an infant being pulled from the birth canal by an extended arm above the head)

4. De Quervain's tenosynovitis: (T/F)
a) Involves the tendon of extensor pollicis longus (F-extensor pollicis brevis is involved)
b) Involves the tendon of abductor pollicis longus (T)
c) Finkelstein's test is part of the standard examination (T)
d) Surgery is needed in most cases (F-most cases resolve with splintage. Sometimes steroid injections are neccesary)

5. Teres major: (T/F)
a) Is a lateral rotator of the humerus (F-it is a medial rotator of the humerus)
b) It contributes to extension of the arm at the shoulder (T-it assists latissimus dorsi in extending the arm)
c) It is supplied by the superior subscapular nerve (F-it is supplied by the inferior subscapular nerve which is a branch of the posterior cord of the brachial plexus)
d) It inserts into the medial lip of the bicipital groove of the humerus (T-teres major originates from the posterior aspect of the inferior scapular border)

6. The lumbricals: (T/F)
a) Extend the metacarpophalangeal joints (F)
b) Flex the metacarpophalangeal joints (T)
c) Extend the interphalangeal joints (T)
d) Flex the interphalangeal joints (F)

7. Regarding serratus anterior: (T/F)
a) It inserts into the lateral border of the scapula (F-the insertion is into the medial scapular border)

b) Its origin is the upper 8 or 9 ribs (T-there is some individual variation, but the origin is always the upper 8 or 9 ribs)
c) It is supplied in part by the medial thoracic artery (F-it is supplied in part by the lateral thoracic artery, which arises from the axillary artery)
d) It is supplied by the long thoracic nerve (T-the long thoracic nerve arises by three roots from the 5th, 6th and 7th cervical nerves (the 7th root may be absent in some individuals)

The branches of the axillary artery are:
From 1st part (medial to pectoralis minor): Superior thoracic artery
From 2nd part (lies behind pectoralis minor): Thoracoacromial artery and lateral thoracic artery
From 3rd part (lateral to pectoralis minor): Subscapular artery, posterior circumflex, anterior circumflex

8. The acromioclavicular joint: (T/F)
a) Derives its stability from 4 ligaments (F-the joint is stabilised by the acromioclavicular ligament, the coracoacromial ligament and the coracoclavicular ligament. The coracoclavicular ligament is made of 2 separate ligaments, the conoid ligament and the trapezoid ligament)
b) Is a synovial joint (T)
c) A grade 3 dislocation of the AC joint involves disruption of the acromioclavicular and coracoclavicular ligaments (T-dislocation of the acromioclavicular joint is graded 1 to 6. Grade 1 injuries involve stretching of the ligaments, but no tear. Grade 2 injuries involve complete tearing of the acromioclavicular ligament and disruption of the coracoacromial ligament. Grade 3 injuries involve complete tears of the acromioclavicular and coracoacromial ligaments. Grades 4 to 6 are variations of

grades 1 to 3 that are are less common but more severe, often requiring surgery)
d) Subacromial impingement rarely involves night pain, waking the patient from sleep (F-night pain is a common symptom, occurring as patients turn in their sleep)

9. The brachial plexus: (T/F)
a) Has 6 roots (F-there are 5 roots, derived from the anterior rami of C5 toT1)
b) Has 3 trunks (T-the superior trunk, derived from C5 and 6, the middle trunk derived from C7 and the inferior trunk derived from C8 and T1)
c) Has 6 divisions (T-the anterior and posterior divisions of the upper, middle, and lower trunks)
d) Has 4 cords (F-there are 3 cords which are named by their position with respect to the axillary artery: The posterior cord is formed from the 3 posterior divisions of the trunks (C5 to T1) The lateral cord is the anterior divisions from the upper and middle trunks (C5 to C7) The medial cord is the continuation of the anterior division of the lower trunk (C8 to T1))

10. Opponens pollicis: (T/F)
a) Is supplied by the ulnar nerve (F-it is innervated by the median nerve)
b) Lies medial to flexor pollicis brevis (F-it lies lateral to flexor pollicis brevis)
c) Inserts into the base of the thumb metacarpal only (F-it is inserted into the whole length of the thumb metacarpal)
d) Originates in part from the flexor retinaculum (T)

11. Regarding the scapula: (T/F)
a) Scapular fracture can be regarded as a 'minor injury' (F-scapular fractures require a significant amount of energy to be transfered to the bone. Scapular fractures are associated with significant thoracic injuries)

b) Winging of the scapula is commonly caused by serratus anterior palsy (F-this is very uncommon. Winging of the scapula is characteristically due to damage to the long thoracic nerve)
c) It is stationary during movements of the shoulder (F-the scapulothoracic articulation is an important part of shoulder and upper limb movements)
d) The superior border of the scapula is palpable (F-the acromion process, the tip of the coracoid process, the spine and inferior border can be palpated, but not the superior border)

12. The biceps: (T/F)
a) Are supplied by the brachial artery (T)
b) Are innervated by the brachial nerve (F-it is supplied by the musculocutaneous nerve. There is no such thing as the brachial nerve!)
c) The brachial pulse is palpated laterally to the biceps tendon (F-the brachial pulsation is medial to the biceps tendon)
d) Tears of the short head of biceps are more common than tears of the long head (F-tears of the long head are more common)

13. The 'triangle of safety' is bounded by the following: (T/F)
a) Anterior border of latissimus dorsi (T)
b) Anterior border of serratus anterior (F)
c) Lateral border of the pectoralis major muscle (T)
d) 5th intercostal space (T)

14. The brachial artery: (T/F)
a) Is the continuation of the axillary artery commencing at the upper border of teres major (F-it commences at the lower border of teres major)
b) Has only the radial artery as a terminal branch (F-the

ulnar artery is also a terminal branch)
c) Lies deep at the elbow (F-it is easily palpated at the elbow, medial to the biceps tendon)
d) Lies lateral to the median nerve in the cubital fossa (T)

15. The median nerve: (T/F)
a) Is the only nerve running through the carpal tunnel (T)
b) Injury at the wrist would result in a 'clawed hand' (T-median nerve damage at the wrist causes a characteristic clawed deformity referred to as 'the hand of benediction'. It is distinct from the 'claw hand' seen in ulnar nerve injury)
c) Supplies all the flexor muscles of the forearm (F-flexor carpi ulnaris and part of flexor digitorum profundus are supplied by the ulnar nerve)
d) Injury to the median nerve causes loss of thumb opposition (T-opposition and flexion of the thumb are lost)

16. Regarding supraspinatus: (T/F)
a) It originates from the spine of the scapula (F-the origin is from the supraspinous fossa of the scapula)
b) It is innervated by the superior subscapular nerve (F-it is supplied by the suprascapular nerve, a branch of the superior trunk derived from C5 and 6)
c) It is supplied by the suprascapular artery (T-the suprascapular artery is a branch of the thyrocervical trunk, which is a branch of the subclavian artery)
d) It is a rotator of the humerus (F-its action is abduction of the humerus and it also contributes to the stability of the shoulder joint as part of the rotator cuff)

17. Regarding the triceps: (T/F)
a) All 3 heads originate from the posterior humerus (F-the long head originates from the infraglenoid tubercle of the scapula, the medial and lateral heads arise from the

posterior humerus)
b) They are innervated by the radial nerve (T-there is also some evidence that the long head has a supply from the axillary artery)
c) Their only action is extension at the elbow (F-the long head contributes to abduction at the shoulder)
d) They are supplied by a branch of the brachial artery (T-it is supplied by the profunda brachii)

18. The radial nerve: (T/F)
a) Has no sensory supply to the hand (F-it supplies a part of the dorsum of the hand. The exact portion of the hand supplied varies between individuals)
b) It arises from the roots of C5 to T1 (T-it arises from the posterior cord, which takes supply from C5 to T1)
c) Radial nerve damage can cause wrist drop (T-the radial nerve supplies the extensors of the forearm. Loss of radial innervation would lead to inability to extend the wrist)
d) Atraumatic radial nerve damage is always permanent (F-atraumatic radial nerve damage is normally transient. Treatment with splintage and physiotherapy usually results in a good functional outcome)

19. The medial epicondyle of the elbow: (T/F)
a) Is the common extensor origin (F-it is the common flexor origin)
b) Has the ulnar nerve running anteriorly (F-the ulnar nerve runs in a groove posterior to the epicondyle)
c) Is inflamed in 'tennis elbow' (F-medial epicondylitis is referred to as 'golfers elbow', lateral epicondylitis is 'tennis elbow')
d) Ossification of the medial epicondyle begins before the lateral epicondyle (F-ossification begins in the medial epicondyle around 6 to 8 years of age, and in the lateral around 13 to 14 years)

The mnemonic CRITOL(E) assists in remembering ossification centres:
Capitellum - 1 year
Radial head - 5 years
Internal (medial) epicondyle - 7 years
Trochlea - 9 years
Olecranon - 11 years
External (lateral) epicondyle : 13 years

20. The axillary nerve: (T/F)
a) When damaged, causes problems with shoulder adduction (F-damage to the axillary nerve causes weakness of deltoid which leads to difficulty abducting)
b) Directly supplies the skin overlying the deltoid (F-the 'regimental badge' area is supplied by the lateral brachial cutaneous nerve, a branch of the axillary nerve)
c) Lies in the triangular space (F-it lies in the quadrangular space)
d) Contributes to the innervation of triceps (T-the long head is supplied by the axillary nerve. The rest of triceps is supplied by the radial nerve)

21. Flexor carpi ulnaris: (T/F)
a) Originates exclusively from the medial epicondyle (F-flexor carpi ulnaris has 2 heads. The ulnar head originates at the medial margin of the olecranon and from the upper two-thirds of the dorsal border of the ulna by an aponeurosis)
b) Inserts to the distal ulna (F-it inserts into the pisiform)
c) The ulnar artery lies medial to flexor carpi ulnaris at the wrist (F-in the anatomical position, the ulnar artery is lateral to flexor carpi ulnaris)
d) Is supplied by the ulnar nerve (T)

22. Flexor pollicis longus: (T/F)
a) Inserts to the base of the proximal phalanx of the

thumb (F-it inserts to the base of the distal phalanx of the thumb)
b) The tendon of flexor pollicis longus runs through the carpal tunnel (T)
c) It is innervated by the ulnar nerve (F-it is innervated by the anterior interosseous nerve, a branch of the median nerve)
d) Has a role in wrist flexion (T-when the thumb is fixed, it assists in flexing the wrist)

23. Flexor carpi radialis: (T/F)
a) Originates from the medial epicondyle (T)
b) Inserts into the hook of the hamate (F-it inserts into the base of the index and middle finger metacarpals)
c) Is supplied by the radial nerve (F-it is supplied by the median nerve)
d) Its action is limited to wrist flexion (F-it is also an abductor of the wrist)

24. The radial artery: (T/F)
a) Arises in the cubital fossa (T-the radial artery arises from the bifurcation of the brachial artery in the cubital fossa)
b) Is the main contributor to the superficial palmar arch (F-the ulnar artery is the main contributor the the superficial palmar arch, with the radial artery contributing via its superficial palmar branch. In some people, the superficial palmar arch is formed entirely from the ulnar artery, with no radial arterial contribution)
c) Is easily palpable at the wrist in patients with a systolic blood pressure of less than 70mmHg (F-a BMJ study, (*Deakin CD, Low JL. BMJ 2000;321:673*) suggests that the presence of a radial pulse indicates the systolic blood pressure is likely to be over 70mmHg)
d) If damaged, can lead to aneurysm formation (T-these

can be iatrogenic e.g. as a result of arterial puncture or cannulation)

25. The ulnar artery: (T/F)
a) Arises directly from the axillary artery (F-it arises form the brachial artery in the cubital fossa)
b) Patency can be checked by Neer's test (F-Allen's test determine adequacy of the ulnar blood supply)
c) Terminates in the deep palmar arch (F-it terminates in the superficial palmar arch)
d) Lies deep to the flexor retinaculum (F-it lies on the flexor retinaculum)

26. Brachialis: (T/F)
a) Is an extender of the elbow (F-it assists biceps in elbow flexion)
b) Is supplied by the radial nerve (T-coracobrachialis, brachialis and biceps are supplied by the musculocutaneous nerve. However the brachialis also receives some fibres from the radial nerve)
c) Contributes to pronation and supination (F-brachialis has no radial insertion and so does not have a role in pronation and supination)
d) Isolated brachialis injuries are common (F-these injuries are rare)

27. The lateral epicondyle of the elbow: (T/F)
a) Is the common extensor origin (T)
b) Is inflamed in tennis elbow (T)
c) Gives rise to the radial collateral ligament (T)
d) Is the origin of pronator teres (F-it is the origin of supinator)

28. Extensor digitorum: (T/F)
a) Arises from the lateral epicondyle of the humerus (T)
b) Has insertions to all 5 digits (F-it has no insertion in the

thumb)
c) Its principle action is on the proximal phalanges (T-the middle and terminal phalanges are extended mainly by the interossei and lumbricals)
d) It is supplied by the anterior interosseous nerve (F-it is supplied by the dorsal interosseous nerve, the continuation of the deep branch of the radial nerve)

29. The cephalic vein: (T/F)
a) Lies medially in the arm (F-the basilic vein is medial)
b) Communicates with the basilic vein (T-via the median cubital vein)
c) Is a good site for large bore venous cannulation (T-it lies superficially and is often visible, allowing relatively easy cannulation)
d) Drains into the basilic vein (F-it drains into the axillary vein, as does the basilic vein)

30. The anatomical snuff box: (T/F)
a) Is bounded by the tendon of extensor pollicis brevis (F-extensor pollicis longus forms the posterior border)
b) Has the radial styloid as its proximal border (T)
c) Has a blood supply which enters distally (T-it is this characteristic that renders the scaphoid at risk of avascular necrosis)
d) Has the median nerve as one of its contents (F-the radial nerve runs through the anatomical snuff box)

31. The deltoid muscle: (T/F)
a) Is supplied by the axillary nerve (T)
b) Its function can be damaged following breast surgery (T-clearance of axillary lymph nodes can cause axillary nerve damage)
c) It is supplied directly by the axillary artery (F-it is supplied by the posterior circumflex artery, which is a branch of the axillary artery)

d) Is the main abductor of the humerus at the shoulder (T- the deltoid is the main abductor of the humerus. Supraspinatus contributes during the first 1 to1500 of abduction; deltoid subsequently acts as the main abductor with supraspinatus contributing towards joint stability)

32. Abductor pollicis brevis: (T/F)
a) Can be palpated in the thenar eminence (T)
b) Is innervated by the ulnar nerve (F-it is innervated by the median nerve)
c) Draws the thumb forward in a plane at right angles to that of the palm of the hand (T-this is abduction in the anatomical position)
d) Inserts into the base of the thumb metacarpal (F-it inserts into the base of the proximal phalanx of the thumb)

33. The quadrangular space: (T/F)
a) Has teres major as one of its boundaries (T)
b) Has the humerus as one of its boundaries (T)
c) Contains the axillary artery (F-it contains the posterior circumflex (humeral) vessels and the axillary nerve)
d) Can be damaged in posterior shoulder dislocations (F-it can be damaged in anterior shoulder dislocations, as the humeral head can compress the posterior circumflex vessels and the axillary nerve)

34. The contents of the carpal tunnel include: (T/F)
a) The tendon of flexor digitorum profundus (T)
b) The radial nerve (F-the median nerve passes through the carpal tunnel)
c) The tendon of flexor pollicis longus (T)
d) The tendon of flexor digitorum superficialis (T)

The contents of the carpal tunnel are:
The tendons of flexor digitorum profundus
The tendons of flexor digitorum superficialis
The tendon of flexor pollicis longus
The median nerve

35. Regarding the interossei of the hand: (T/F)
a) There are 3 dorsal interossei (F-there are 4 dorsal interossei)
b) There are 3 palmar interossei (T)
c) They are supplied by the ulnar nerve (T)
d) The dorsal interossei abduct the fingers away from the middle finger (T-the palmar interossei adduct the fingers towards the little finger)

36. Regarding latissimus dorsi: (T/F)
a) It is supplied by a branch of the subscapular artery (T-latissimus dorsi is supplied by the thoracodorsal branch of the subscapular artery which in turn is the largest branch of the axillary artery)
b) It is an external rotator of the arm (F-latissimus dorsi adducts, extends and internally rotates the arm)
c) It inserts into the humerus (T-it inserts into the floor of the intertubercular groove of the humerus)
d) It is supplied by a branch of the posterior cord of the brachial plexus (T-it is supplied by the thoracodorsal nerve, which is derived from the ventral rami of the 6th, 7th and 8th cervical nerves)

37. The ulnar nerve: (T/F)
a) Can be directly damaged following a fracture of the humerus (T-the ulnar nerve originates from the C8 to T1 nerve roots which form part of the medial cord of the brachial plexus and descends on the posteromedial aspect of the humerus)
b) Runs through the carpal tunnel (F-the median nerve is

the only nerve to run through the carpal tunnel)
c) Is medial to the ulnar artery at the wrist (T-this orientation is particularly important when considering ulnar nerve blocks)
d) Is derived from the posterior cord of the brachial plexus (F-it is derived from the medial cord of the brachial plexus)

38. Regarding trapezius: (T/F)
a) Its origin includes the nuchal ligament (T)
b) It inserts into the wing of the scapula (F-the insertions are the posterior border of the lateral third of the clavicle, acromion process and spine of the scapula)
c) Its innervation is via the dorsal rami of C3 and C4 (F-the innervation is from the accessory nerve, and the ventral rami of C3 and C4)
d) It is innervated by a branch of the thyrocervical trunk (T-the transverse cervical artery is a branch of the thyrocervical trunk, which in turn is a branch of the subclavian artery)

39. Regarding forearm fractures: (T/F)
a) A Monteggia fracture is a fracture of the ulna with dislocation of the radial head (T)
b) A Galeazzi fracture a fracture of the ulna with dislocation of the distal radioulnar joint (F-the fracture involved is an ulnar fracture)
c) A Barton's fracture is a distal radius fracture with dislocation of the radiocarpal joint (T)
d) A Smith's fracture is a distal radius fracture with dorsal displacement of the distal fracture segment (F-a Smith's fracture has volar displacement of the distal fracture segment. A Colles fracture has dorsal displacement of the distal fracture segment)

40. Subscapularis: (T/F)
a) Arises from the subscapular fossa (T)
b) Inserts into the greater tubercle of the humerus (F-the insertion is to the lesser tubercle of the humerus)
c) Is supplied by branches of the lateral cord of the brachial plexus (F-subscapularis is supplied by the superior and inferior subscapular nerves, which are branches of the posterior cord of the brachial plexus and are derived from C5 and C6)
d) It medially rotates the humerus (T-it also contributes to the stabilisation of the shoulder joint)

LOWER LIMB ANSWERS

1. Flexor hallucis longus: (T/F)
a) Is a plantar flexor of the foot (T-it flexes all the joints of the great toe as well as plantar flexing the foot at the ankle joint)
b) Inserts into the base of the proximal phalanx of the great toe (F-it inserts into the base of the distal phalanx)
c) Is supplied by the tibial nerve (T)
d) Contributes to being able to stand on tip-toes (T-flexor digitorum longus and flexor hallucis longus are the direct flexors of the phalanges; they also extend (plantar flex) the foot upon the leg. They assist gastrocnemius and soleus in extending the foot, as in the act of walking, or in standing on tiptoe)

2. Sartorius: (T/F)
a) Is the longest muscle in the human body (T)
b) Originates from the anterior superior iliac spine (T)
c) Contributes to knee flexion (T)
d) Is innervated by the sciatic nerve (F-it is innervated by the femoral nerve)

3. Biceps femoris: (T/F)
a) Is an extender of the hip joint (T-the long head contributes to extension of the hip)
b) Is innervated by branches of the sciatic nerve (T-the short head of the biceps femoris is innervated by the common peroneal branch of the sciatic nerve, while the long head is innervated by the tibial branch of the sciatic nerve)
c) Arises entirely within the pelvis (F-the short head of biceps femoris arises from the linea aspera of the femur)
d) Inserts only into the fibula (F-the muscle inserts into the lateral side of the head of the fibula, and also into the lateral condyle of the tibia)

4. The medial collateral ligament: (T/F)
a) Originates from the medial epicondyle of the femur (T)
b) Inserts into the medial condyle of the tibia (T)
c) Is characteristically damaged by a varus injury (F-it is characteristically injured by a valgus stress, e.g. a football player being kicked on the lateral side of the knee)
d) Has a insertion into the medial meniscus (T-the medial collateral ligament has an insertion into the medial meniscus, but the lateral collateral has no such insertion)

5. Regarding hip adduction: (T/F)
a) The majority of the hip adductors are supplied by the obturator nerve (T-the obturator nerve is responsible for the motor innervation of the external obturator, adductor longus, adductor brevis, adductor magnus, gracilis and has an inconsistent supply to pectineus)
b) The hip adductors originate from the pubic ramus and symphysis (T)
c) The hip adductors are supplied by the L2 to L4 nerves (T-via the obturator nerves)
d) The obturator nerve has a sensory supply to the anterior thigh (F-the obturator nerve supplies the medial thigh)

6. Peroneus brevis: (T/F)
a) Is supplied by the tibial artery (F-it is supplied by the peroneal artery, a branch of the posterior tibial artery)
b) Is a plantar flexor of the foot (T-it also everts the foot)
c) Can cause an avulsion fracture of the base of the 5th metatarsal if over-stretched (T)
d) Is supplied by the deep peroneal nerve (F-it is supplied by the superficial peroneal nerve)

7. The femoral artery: (T/F)
a) Arises directly from the external iliac artery (T-the common femoral artery arises from the external iliac

artery behind the inguinal ligament. It subsequently gives off deep and superficial branches, the profunda femoris and superficial femoral artery respectively)
b) The superficial femoral artery supplies the thigh (F-the thigh is supplied by the profunda femoris)
c) Contributes a supply to the genitals (T-via the deep and superficial external pudendal arteries)
d) Becomes the popliteal artery in the adductor hiatus (T-the femoral vessels become the popliteal vessels as they leave the adductor hiatus)

8. The great saphenous vein: (T/F)
a) Is visible over the lateral malleolus of the ankle (F-it is visible over the medial malleolus, where it can be useful for venous access)
b) Drains into the external iliac vein (F-it joins with the femoral vein at the saphenofemoral junction)
c) When thrombosed, constitutes a deep venous thrombosis (F-the great saphenous vein is a superficial vein and hence cannot be considered a deep venous thrombosis when thrombosed)
d) Is a common site of varicose veins (T)

9. Regarding lymph nodes: (T/F)
a) The superficial inguinal lymph nodes are situated above the inguinal ligament (F-the superficial inguinal lymph nodes form a chain immediately below the inguinal ligament)
b) Cloquet's node is found in the deep inguinal lymph nodes (T)
c) The deep inguinal lymph nodes drain into the external iliac lymph nodes (T)
d) The external iliac lymph nodes drain directly into the para-aortic lymph nodes (F-the external iliac lymph nodes drain into the common iliac lymph nodes, which then drain into the lateral aortic lymph nodes)

10. The following are components of the deltoid ligament of the ankle joint: (T/F)
a) Calcaneotibial ligament (T)
b) Anterior talotibial (T)
c) Posterior talocalcaneal ligament (F)
d) Medial talocalcaneal ligament (F)

The deltoid ligament *(otherwise known as the medial ligament of the talocrural joint), is a flat triangular band which attaches to the medial malleolus. It is comprised of the anterior tibiotalar ligament, the tibiocalcaneal ligament, the posterior tibiotalar ligament, and the tibionavicular Ligament. These are arranged in two layers, superficial and deep*

11. Psoas major: (T/F)
a) Arises from the T12 to L5 vertebrae and their intervertebral discs (T)
b) Inserts into the greater trochanter of the femur (F-it inserts into the lesser trochanter)
c) Is a medial rotator of the thigh (F-it is a lateral rotator of the thigh, as well as a hip flexor)
d) Is innervated by the femoral nerve (F-it is innervated by the lumbar plexus via L1 to L3)

12. The following bones are components of the lateral arch of the foot: (T/F)
a) Calcaneum (T)
b) Cuboid (T)
c) 3rd, 4th and 5th metatarsals (F-the 4th and 5th metatarsals are components of the lateral arch of the foot, the 3rd metatarsal is part of the medial arch)
d) Lateral cuneiform (F-the lateral cuneiform is part of the medial arch)

The lateral arch *is composed of the calcaneum, the cuboid, and the 4th and 5th metatarsals*

13. Regarding the anterior thigh: (T/F)
a) Iliacus is a medial hip rotator (F-Iliacus is a hip flexor and a lateral rotator)
b) Iliacus originates in part from the anterior superior iliac spine (T-Iliacus also arises from the iliac fossa of the pelvis)
c) Pectineus is a medial hip rotator (T-pectineus also flexes and adducts the hip)
d) Pectineus can form the covering of an obturator hernia (T-this form of hernia is more common in women and is an unusual, but important cause of bowel obstruction)

14. The medial meniscus: (T/F)
a) Heals quickly after injury if the injury is to the inner part of the medial meniscus (F-due to its poor blood supply, the inner two-thirds of the medial meniscus is slow to heal. The outer third heals more quickly, hence conservative treatment is more likely to be successful with injuries to the outer part of the medial meniscus)
b) If removed surgically (menisectomy), leads to a higher risk of osteoarthritis (T)
c) If injured, is characteristically injured in isolation (F-it is more common to have associated injuries to the medial collateral ligament and/or the anterior cruciate ligament)
d) Is not involved in the pattern of injury known as O'Donoghue's triad (F-O'Donoghue's triad is the eponym given to a knee injury comprising a medial collateral ligament tear, a medial meniscal injury and an anterior cruciate ligament tear. In athletes sustaining this pattern of injury, there is some evidence to suggest that the lateral meniscus is more commonly injured than the medial meniscus)

15. Rectus Femoris: (T/F)
a) Inserts into the patella (T-it inserts into the patella by the quadriceps tendon)

b) Arises in part from the anterior superior iliac spine (T-the other point of origin is a groove above the brim of the acetabulum)
c) Is supplied by the sciatic nerve (F-it is supplied by the femoral nerve)
d) Is an extender of the knee (T-in addition to flexing the hip, rectus femoris functions as a knee extender. It can perform this action as it arises from the pelvis, unlike the other components of the quadriceps which arise from the femur)

16. The dorsalis pedis artery: (T/F)
a) Is palpable medial to the tendon of extensor hallucis longus (F-the artery is palpable lateral to the tendon of extensor hallucis longus)
b) Is always palpable in young healthy individuals (F-there is evidence that the dorsalis pedis is impalpable in 2 to 3% of young healthy individuals, (*Robertson, GS; Ristic, CD; Bullen, BR (1990). The incidence of congenitally absent foot pulses. Annals of the Royal College of Surgeons of England 72 (2): 99–100*)
c) Is the continuation of the anterior tibial artery (T)
d) Gives off the deep plantar artery (T-the dorsalis pedis divides into 2 branches at the proximal part of the 1st intermetatarsal space; the dorsal metatarsal artery and the deep plantar artery)

17. Damage to the common peroneal nerve: (T/F)
a) Can be caused by a Maisonneuve fracture (T-a Maisonneuve fracture includes a fracture of the head of the fibula, which has the common peroneal nerve adjacent to it)
b) Can cause foot-drop (T)
c) Can cause sensory loss on the dorsum of the foot (T-the cutaneous innervation of the dorsum of the foot is via the deep and superficial peroneal nerves. Both are branches

of the common peroneal nerve)
d) Can cause sensory loss over the heel (F-the cutaneous innervation of the heel is via the tibial nerve)

18. The following landmarks are components of the Ottawa ankle & foot rule: (T/F)
a) Lateral malleolus (T)
b) Calcaneum (F)
c) Navicular (T)
d) Base of 5th metatarsal (T)

The 'Ottawa landmarks' are the medial and lateral malleoli, the navicular and the base of the 5th metatarsal

19. Regarding lower limb compartment syndrome: (T/F)
a) Loss of peripheral pulses is an early sign (F-pulses are only affected if the relevant arteries are contained within the affected compartment due to the pressures that cause compartment syndrome often being well below arterial pressures. This allows arterial flow to persist in many cases)
b) Pain is an early sign (T-pain is the most consistent early sign. It is severe, often poorly localised and characteristically out of proportion to the injury sustained)
c) It is always related to trauma (F-there are numerous non-traumatic causes of lower limb compartment syndrome e.g. intravenous drug use and long periods spent in the lithotomy position as in gynaecological surgery)
d) Rhabdomyolysis is a known consequence (T)

20. The patellar tendon: (T/F)
a) Inserts into the tibia tuberosity (T)
b) When inflamed, along with its insertion, is known as Kohler's syndrome (F-Osgood–Schlatter syndrome is

traction apophysitis of the patellar tendon and the tibial tuberosity. Kohler's syndrome is traction apophysitis of the navicular)
c) When ruptured, leads to an inability to straight leg raise (T)
d) Has a bursa posterior to it (F-The posterior surface of the patellar ligament is separated from the synovial membrane of the joint by a large infrapatellar pad. It is separated from the tibia by a bursa, which can become inflamed, causing infrapatellar bursitis)

21. Regarding vastus lateralis: (T/F)
a) It originates in part from gluteus maximus (T)
b) It inserts only into the patella (F-it also inserts into the capsule of the knee joint)
c) It is a lateral rotator of the hip (F-the quadriceps are knee extenders and contribute to the stability of the knee joint)
d) It is supplied by the femoral artery (T)

22. The acetabulum: (T/F)
a) Is formed from the united pubis, ischium and ilium (T-the bony components of the pelvis unite to form the acetabulum)
b) Is orientated posteriorly (F-it is orientated anteriorly, downwardly and laterally)
c) Has a uniformly sized labrum surrounding it (F-the labrum is irregularly sized)
d) The labrum is extracapsular (F-the 2 surfaces of the labrum are covered by synovial membrane, the external one being in contact with the capsule, the internal one being inclined inward, which narrows the acetabulum. The inner layer embraces the cartilaginous surface of the head of the femur)

23. The femoral nerve (T/F)
a) Arises from the 2nd to 4th lumbar nerves (T)
b) Innervates the skin on the posterior aspect of the thigh (F-the sciatic nerve innervates the skin on the posterior aspect of the thigh and gluteal regions)
c) Runs through the femoral canal (F-the femoral canal contains lymphatic vessels and Cloquet's nodes only)
d) Supplies the quadriceps (T)

24. The ligamentum teres: (T/F)
a) Blends with the transverse acetabular ligament (T)
b) Attaches to the inferior surface of the fovea of the head of the femur (F-the ligamentum teres implants into the antero-superior part of the fovea)
c) Contributes significantly to the stability of the hip joint (F-the ligamentum teres has little, if any, influence upon the mechanism of the joint)
d) Transmits a branch of the femoral nerve to the hip joint (F-it transmits a branch of the posterior branch of the obturator artery)

25. The saphenous nerve: (T/F)
a) Passes through the femoral triangle (T)
b) Is a branch of the femoral nerve (T-the saphenous nerve is the largest cutaneous branch of the femoral nerve)
c) Supplies the skin on the lateral part of the lower leg (F-most of the sensory supply of the lower leg is from the sciatic nerve. The saphenous nerve supplies the skin on the medial part of the lower leg)
d) Is not at risk of damage during cutdown of the long saphenous vein (F-this is a known complication of venous cutdown)

26. Adductor longus: (T/F)
a) Is a flexor of the hip (T-in addition to adduction, adductor longus is a weak hip flexor)
b) Originates from the anterior superior iliac spine (F-it originates from the body of the pubic bone)
c) Is supplied by the femoral nerve (F-it is supplied by the anterior branch of the obturator nerve)
d) Forms the medial wall of the femoral triangle (T)

27. Obturator externus
a) Is a lateral rotator of the hip (T-as well as adducting the hip, obturator externus rotates the thigh laterally)
b) Is a medial rotator of the hip (F-obturator externus rotates the thigh laterally)
c) Is supplied by the femoral nerve (F-it is supplied by the obturator nerve)
d) Inserts into the trochanteric fossa of the femur (T)

28. The obturator nerve: (T/F)
a) Supplies the skin on the anterior surface of the thigh (F-the obturator nerve supplies the medial side of the thigh. The anterior surface of the thigh is supplied by cutaneous branches of the femoral nerve)
b) Supplies all the hip adductors (T)
c) Passes through the obturator canal (T-the obturator artery and vein, as well as the obturator nerve, all travel through the obturator canal)
d) Has an accessory obturator nerve in approximately one-third of cases (T)

29. Regarding the gluteal muscles: (T/F)
a) Gluteus maximus inserts into the femur (T-it inserts into the gluteal tuberosity of the femur)
b) They are supplied by the sciatic nerve (F-they are supplied by the superior gluteal nerve)
c) A positive Trendelenberg sign can indicate gluteal

injury or paralysis (T)
d) Gluteus maximus acts as a medial hip rotator (F-it acts as a lateral rotator of the hip)

30. Peroneus longus: (T/F)
a) Plantar flexes the foot (T-it also everts the foot)
b) Causes avulsion fractures of the base of the 5th metatarsal when over-stretched (F-the tendon of peroneus longus crosses the sole of the foot obliquely and inserts into the 1st metatarsal and the medial cuneiform. The tendon of peroneus brevis inserts into the base of the 5th metatarsal and can cause avulsion fractures)
c) Is supplied by the deep peroneal nerve (F-it is supplied by the superficial peroneal nerve)
d) Is in the anterior compartment of the lower leg (F-it is in the lateral compartment)

31. The sciatic nerve: (T/F)
a) Arises from the lumbo-sacral plexus (T-the sciatic nerve is formed from the L4 to S3 spinal nerves)
b) Gives off the deep peroneal nerve as a direct branch (F-the deep peroneal nerve is a branch of the common peroneal nerve, which is a branch of the sciatic nerve)
c) Can be damaged by intra-muscular injections into the buttocks (T-intramuscular injections into the buttocks should be given into the 'upper and outer' quadrant, to avoid the sciatic nerve which runs more medially)
d) Can be damaged by hip dislocation (T-posterior hip dislocation can cause sciatic nerve injury. This injury is uncommon and characteristically follows high energy impacts such as high speed road traffic collisions)

32. Tibialis anterior: (T/F)
a) Is situated medial to the tibia (F-it lies lateral to the tibia)
b) Originates from the tibial tuberosity (F-it originates

from the lateral condyle and upper part of the lateral tibia. It also originates from the adjoining part of the interosseous membrane and from the deep surface of the fascia)
c) Is an inverter of the foot (T-it also dorsiflexes the foot)
d) Is supplied by the deep peroneal nerve (T)

33. The semitendinosus muscle: (T/F)
a) Has a short tendon at its attachment (F-the tendon is notably long)
b) Inserts into the posterior surface of the tibia (F-it inserts into the upper part of the medial surface of the body of the tibia. The insertion is carried on anteriorly rather than posteriorly)
c) Has an insertion into the medial collateral ligament of the knee (F-the tendon of semitendinosus passes over the medial collateral ligament of the knee and is separated from the medial collateral ligament by a bursa)
d) Is supplied by the sciatic nerve (T-it is supplied by muscular branches of the sciatic nerve)

34. Extensor hallucis longus: (T/F)
a) Extends the little toe (F-it extends the great toe as well as assisting with foot dorsiflexion and inversion)
b) Is supplied by the tibial nerve (F-it is supplied by the deep peroneal nerve)
c) Inserts into the base of the distal phalanx of the great toe (T)
d) Is separated from tibialis anterior by the anterior tibial vessels and deep peroneal nerve (T-the anterior tibial vessels and deep peroneal nerve lie between extensor hallucis longus and tibialis anterior)

35. The popliteal fossa: (T/F)
a) Has the tendons of semimembranosus and semitendinosus as its medial superior border (T)

b) Has vastus intermedialis as its lateral superior border (F-the tendon of biceps femoris is the lateral superior border)
c) Has the medial head of gastrocnemius as the medial inferior border (T)
d) Has plantaris only as its lower lateral border (F-the lateral head of gastrocnemius is also part of the lateral inferior border)

36. Regarding the plantar calcaneonavicular ligament ('spring ligament')
a) Its calcaneal origin is at the sustentaculum tali (T-the plantar calcaneonavicular ligament connects the sustentaculum tali of the calcaneus to the plantar surface of the navicular)
b) It is not connected to the deltoid ligament (F-its medial border is blended with the forepart of the deltoid ligament)
c) It is significantly involved in supporting the arch of the foot (T-by supporting the head of the talus, the plantar calcaneonavicular ligament contributes to maintaining the arch of the foot)
d) It has tibialis anterior inserting into its dorsal surface (F-the tendon of the tibialis posterior supports the ligament on its plantar surface)

37. The contents of the popliteal fossa include: (T/F)
a) The common peroneal nerve (F-the common peroneal nerve descends obliquely along the lateral side of the popliteal fossa and then to the fibular head)
b) The tibial nerve (T)
c) The popliteal artery (T)
d) The popliteal vein (T)

38. A patient presents to the Emergency Department after sustaining an inversion injury to his right ankle the

previous night. He has no tenderness at any of the 'Ottawa points' and can mobilise. He has a specific area of tenderness and swelling anterior to the lateral malleolus. The single most likely structure to have been injured is the: (T/F)
a) Calcaneofibular ligament (F-isolated injuries to the calcaneofibular ligament are unusual)
b) Lateral malleolus (F-apart from a small avulsion fracture, the lateral malleolus is unlikely to be injured as the malleolus is not focally tender)
c) Anterior talofibular ligament (T-this ligament is commonly injured in ankle sprains)
d) Posterior talofibular ligament (F-the presence of swelling anterior to the lateral malleolus would suggest the anterior talofibular ligament is more likely to be injured in this situation)

39. Popliteus: (T/F)
a) Is a flexor of the knee (T)
b) Has a relatively unimportant role in knee movements (F-it is a very important muscle. Popliteus produces the slight medial rotation of the tibia, which is essential in the early stage of knee flexion. Popliteus also has a role in protecting the lateral meniscus during flexion. It is attached to the lateral meniscus and draws the meniscus posteriorly during knee flexion. This prevents crushing of the meniscus between the tibia and femur as the knee flexes)
c) Is supplied by the tibial nerve (T)
d) Is supplied by the tibial artery (F-it is supplied by the popliteal artery)

40. The posterior tibial artery: (T/F)
a) Gives off the peroneal artery in the popliteal fossa (F-there is some variation in the site of the origin of the peroneal artery but the posterior tibial artery typically

gives off the peroneal artery approximately 2.5 cm below the lower border of the popliteus)
b) Is palpable anterior to the medial malleolus (F-the posterior tibial artery pulsation is palpable posterior to the medial malleolus)
c) Is impalpable in 2 to 3% of healthy adults (F-it is more consistently palpable than the dorsalis pedis, being impalpable in approximately 0.2% of healthy individuals, (Robertson, GS; Ristic, CD; Bullen, BR (1990). *The incidence of congenitally absent foot pulses. Annals of the Royal College of Surgeons of England 72 (2): 99-100*)
d) Supplies the sole of the foot (T-via the medial and lateral plantar arteries)

41. Anterior cruciate ligament tears: (T/F)
a) Can be diagnosed using McMurray's test (F-McMurray's test is used to detect meniscal injuries. The Lachman or anterior drawer test is used in the diagnosis of anterior cruciate ligament injuries)
b) Are often asymptomatic (F-the injury results in pain and swelling of the knee and patients often report a 'popping' sound or sensation at the time of the injury)
c) Always need reconstructive surgery in athletes (F-physiotherapy focusing on strengthening the quadriceps and hamstring can have very favourable results, even in athletes)
d) Inserts into the medial and back part of the lateral femoral condyle (T)

42. Regarding the bursae of the knee: (T/F)
a) Inflammation of the pre-patellar bursa is referred to as 'housemaids knee' (T-pre-patellar bursitis is a common cause of anterior knee pain. It is due to inflammation of the prepatellar bursa. It is common in people whose occupation necessitates a lot of kneeling e.g. roofers, plumbers, carpet layers and gardeners)

b) Infrapatellar bursitis is known as 'clergymans knee' (T-infrapatellar bursitis is inflammation of the superficial infrapatellar bursa which is located just below the patella. It has a historical association with clergymen due to kneeling on hard surfaces, e.g. during church services)
c) The deep infrapatellar bursa facilitates movement of the patellar ligament over the tibia (T-the deep infrapatellar bursa lies between the upper part of the tibia and the patellar ligament. It allows for movement of the patellar ligament over the tibia)
d) The fibular bursa lies between the lateral collateral ligament and the tendon of semitendinosus (F-the fibular bursa lies between the lateral collateral ligament and the tendon of the biceps femoris)

43. Femoral nerve damage: (T/F)
a) Can be caused by arterial blood gas sampling from the femoral artery (T-the proximity of the femoral nerve to the artery leaves the nerve vulnerable to damage during procedures involving arterial puncture e.g. arterial blood gas sampling and arterial line insertion)
b) Affects flexion of the hip (T-rectus femoris, which is supplied by the femoral nerve, is a flexor of the hip)
c) Is a relatively common consequence of total hip replacement (F-femoral nerve damage is uncommon following total hip replacement)
d) Can cause a decrease in the knee jerk reflex (T)

44. Tibialis posterior: (T/F)
a) Is in the medial compartment of the calf (F-it is in the posterior compartment of the calf)
b) Inverts the foot (T-it also assists in plantar flexion of the foot)
c) Is supplied by the common peroneal nerve (F-it is supplied by the tibial nerve)
d) Has its primary insertion into the navicular (T-it has

subsequent fibrous expansions; to the sustentaculum tali of the calcaneus, to the 3 cuneiforms, the cuboid, and the bases of the 2nd, 3rd, and 4th metatarsals)

45. The sural nerve: (T/F)
a) Supplies the skin of the heel and lateral hindfoot (T)
b) Can be blocked using subcutaneous infiltration with local anaesthetic posterior to the lateral malleolus (T)
c) Arises solely from the common peroneal nerve (F-the sural nerve arises from the medial sural cutaneous nerve, which is a branch of the tibial nerve, and the lateral sural cutaneous nerve which originates from the common peroneal nerve)
d) Is used for nerve biopsies in the diagnosis of peripheral neuropathies and amyloidosis (T)

46. The following are components of the lateral ligament of the ankle joint: (T/F)
a) Anterior talofibular ligament (T)
b) Calcaneonavicular ligament (F)
c) Calcaneotibial ligament (F)
d) Calcaneofibular ligament (T)

The lateral ligament of the ankle joint is comprised of the anterior talofibular ligament, the posterior talofibular ligament and the calcaneofibular ligament

47. The obturator nerve: (T/F)
a) Is derived from the first 3 lumbar nerves (F-the obturator nerve is derived from the L2 to L4 spinal nerves)
b) Innervates the skin on the medial aspect of the thigh (T)
c) Innervates the obturator internus muscle (F-obturator internus, a hip abductor and lateral rotator, is supplied by the nerve to obturator internus, which originates in the sacral plexus. It arises from the ventral divisions of the

5th lumbar and 1st and 2nd sacral nerves)
d) Supplies the majority of the hip adductors (T-the obturator nerve is responsible for the motor innervation of the external obturator, adductor longus, adductor brevis, adductor magnus and gracilis. It also has an inconsistent supply to pectineus)

48. Regarding the subtalar joint: (T/F)
a) It is comprised of the junction between the talus and the calcaneum (T)
b) Does not contribute to dorsi- and plantar flexion of the foot (F-the subtalar joint has a very significant role in facilitating dorsi- and plantar flexion of the foot)
c) Does not have a joint capsule (F-the 2 bones are connected by an articular capsule)
d) Subtalar joint dislocations always involve disruption of the ankle joint (F-the ankle joint is undisturbed in subtalar joint dislocations)

49. The lateral collateral ligament: (T/F)
a) Is wider than the medial collateral ligament (F-the medial collateral ligament is much wider than the lateral collateral)
b) Inserts into the fibular head (T)
c) Is attached to the lateral meniscus (F-the medial collateral ligament has an insertion into the medial meniscus, but the lateral collateral is separated from the lateral meniscus by the popliteus tendon)
d) Originates from the lateral femoral condyle (T)

50. The achilles tendon: (T/F)
a) Is formed by the fibres of gastrocnemius only (F-the soleus also contributes to the achilles tendon)
b) Can be deemed intact if plantar flexion is possible (F-plantar flexion may still be possible if the achilles tendon is ruptured due to the effects of tibialis posterior, the

peroneal muscles and the toe flexors)
c) Is particularly at risk of rupture in patients taking long term steroids (T)
d) Has a bursa between its lower end and the calcaneus (T- the retrocalcaneal bursa lies between the calcaneum and the achilles tendon. Inflammation of this bursa can be mistaken for achilles tendonitis)

HEAD AND NECK ANSWERS

1. Regarding sternocleidomastoid: (T/F)
a) It originates from the sternum only (F sternocleidomastoid originates from the manubrium of the sternum and the medial third of the clavicle)
b) It inserts into the occipital bone (T-as well as inserting into the mastoid process of the temporal bone, sternocleidomastoid inserts into the occipital bone)
c) Its only action is rotation of the head (F-when both the right and left sternocleidomastoid muscles contract, the head is extended and the neck is flexed)
d) Its anterior border covers the carotid arteries (T)

2. The cricothyroid ligament: (T/F)
a) Forms the vocal ligaments (T-the vocal ligaments are formed by the upper margins of the cricothyroid ligament)
b) Can be located inferior to the thryoid cartilage (T-this is how the cricothyroid ligament is located, e.g. when preparing for an emergency cricothyroidotomy)
c) Receives the anterior end of each vocal cord (F-the anterior end of each vocal cord is attached to the thyroid cartilage)
d) Receives the posterior end of each vocal cord (F-the posterior end of each vocal cord attaches to the vocal process of the arytenoid cartilage)

3. Horner's syndrome: (T/F)
a) Causes a dilated pupil (F-the pupil is constricted in Horner's syndrome)
b) Is caused by a deficiency of sympathetic supply to the eye (T)
c) Is associated with increased sweating (F-decreased sweating on the affected side of the face is often seen)
d) Causes total paralysis of the levator palpebrae

superioris (F-levator palpebrae superioris is only partially supplied by the autonomic nervous system. Its smooth muscle has a sympathetic innervation, whereas the striated muscle is controlled by the oculomotor nerve, which is under voluntary control. This explains why patients with Horner's syndrome can partially elevate their eyelids)

4. Enlargement of the pituitary gland is associated with: (T/F)
a) Bilateral nasal visual field defects (F-bilateral temporal visual field defects are seen in pituitary enlargement, due to pressure on the optic chiasm)
b) Sheehan's syndrome (F-This is hypopituitarism due to pituitary necrosis seen following haemorrhage during childbirth)
c) Erosion of the sella turcica (T-this is a part of the sphenoid. When eroded due to pituitary enlargement, the effects can be seen on lateral skull radiographs)
d) Headache (T-any cause of raised intracranial pressure can produce headache)

5. The glossopharyngeal nerve: (T/F)
a) Decends through the skull via the jugular foramen (T)
b) Is entirely sensory (F-it has a motor supply to stylopharyngeus)
c) Contributes to blood pressure control (T-the carotid branch of the glossopharyngeal nerve supplies the carotid sinus and body (along with the vagus and sympathetics) which control blood pressure, heart rate and respiration)
d) Supplies the posterior one-third of the tongue (T-it has sensory supply to the posterior one-third of the tongue. The motor supply is via the hypoglossal nerve)

6. The anterior triangle of the neck: (T/F)
a) Is bounded superiorly by the mandible (T-the anterior

triangle of the neck is bounded superiorly by the body of the mandible)
b) Is bounded anteriorly by the digastric muscle (F-the anterior triangle of the neck is bounded anteriorly by the midline)
c) Is bounded posteriorly by the sternocleidomastoid (T)
d) Has the jugular notch of the manubrium as its apex (T)

7. The medial wall of the orbit is formed by the following bones: (T/F)
a) Frontal process of the maxilla (T)
b) Lacrimal bone (T)
c) Greater wing of the sphenoid (F-the body of the sphenoid forms part of the medial wall of the orbit)
d) Ethmoid (T-the orbital plate of the ethmoid forms part of the medial wall of the orbit)

8. The thyroid gland: (T/F)
a) Has 4 lobes (F-the thyroid gland has 2 lobes, with a narrow isthmus connecting them)
b) Is directly supplied by the carotid artery (F-the thyroid galnd is supplied by the superior and inferior thyroid arteries, which are branches of the external carotid and thyrocervical trunk respectively)
c) Has its venous drainage directly into the internal jugular vein (F-the superior and middle thyroid veins drain into the internal jugular vein. The inferior thyroid vein drains into the left brachiocephalic vein)
d) Has the parathyroid glands posterior to it (T-the 4 parathyroid glands are situated posterior to the thyroid gland. The 2 superior parathyroid glands are posterior to the middle of the thyroid and the 2 inferior parathyroid glands are posterior to the lower part of the thyroid)

9. Regarding the facial vein: (T/F)
a) It communicates with the cavernous sinus (T-the facial

and opthalmic veins communicate with the cavernous sinus. This is a potential route for intracranial transmission of facial infections)
b) It is formed by the union of the superficial temporal and supraorbital veins (F-the facial vein is formed by the union of the supratrochlear and supraorbital veins)
c) It drains into the external jugular vein (F-it drains into the internal jugular vein)
d) It crosses the face above the mandible as it descends (F-it crosses the mandible as it descends toward the internal jugular vein)

10. Clinical signs of a base of skull fracture include: (T/F)
a) Mastoid bruising (T-this indicates a fracture of the petrous temporal bone)
b) Blood in the external ear canal (F-blood in the external ear canal is often the result of bleeding from a scalp wound pooling in the external auditory meatus. A base of skull fracture may be indicated by fluid being visible behind the tympanic membrane, or by seeing blood or CSF oozing through a ruptured tympanic membrane)
c) Bleeding from the nostrils (F-epistaxis is not uncommon following head/face injury. CSF coming from the nostrils (rhinorhoea) is a sign of base of skull fracture)
d) Bilateral orbital ecchymoses (T-in the absence of bilateral facial trauma, this is the 'Panda eyes' sign)

11. Regarding the carotid sheath: (T/F)
a) It is formed from prevertebral fascia only (F-the carotid sheath is formed from the pre-tracheal, the pre-vertebral and the investing layers of deep fascia)
b) It surrounds the external carotid artery (F-the carotid sheath surrounds the common and internal carotid arteries)
c) It surrounds the recurrent laryngeal nerve (F)
d) It surrounds the vagus nerve (T-the carotid sheath

surrounds the common and internal carotid arteries, the vagus nerve, the internal jugular vein and the deep cervical lymph nodes)

12. The oculomotor nerve: (T/F)
a) Enters the orbit through the superior orbital fissure (T- the oculomotor nerve enters the orbit through the superior orbital fissure between the 2 heads of laterus rectus)
b) Supplies all the ocular muscles (F-the oculomotor nerve supplies all the ocular nerves except superior oblique and rectus lateralis)
c) Controls pupillary constriction (T-the oculomotor nerve supplies parasympathetic fibres to the pupillary sphincter which constricts the pupils)
d) Runs along the medial wall of the cavernous sinus (F- the oculomotor nerve
runs along the lateral wall of the cavernous sinus)

13. Regarding scalenus anterior: (T/F)
a) It originates from the 3rd to 6th cervical vertebrae (T- scalenus anterior arises from the transverse processes of the 3rd to 6th cervical vertebrae)
b) It inserts into the medial clavicle (F-it inserts into the 1st rib)
c) It is innervated by the C5 and C6 spinal nerves (T)
d) It is a rotator of the neck (T-scalenus anterior also elevates the 1st rib and laterally flexes the neck)

14. Clinical features of a middle cerebral artery stroke include the following: (T/F)
a) Ipsilateral hemiplegia (F-a contralateral hemiplegia is seen in middle cerebral artery stroke)
b) Eyes deviated toward the side of the infarction (T)
c) Loss of consciousness (T-this is relatively rare, but does occur. It can be due to seizures or raised intracranial

pressure)
d) Contralateral hemianopia (T)

15. The recurrent laryngeal nerve: (T/F)
a) Is a branch of the vagus nerve (T)
b) On the right, runs around the subclavian artery (T-the right recurrent laryngeal nerve 'hooks' around the 1st part of the subclavian artery)
c) Supplies all the muscles of the larynx (F-the recurrent laryngeal nerve supplies all the laryngeal muscles except cricothyroid, which is supplied by the superior laryngeal nerve)
d) If damaged, can cause a hoarse voice (T)

16. The parotid gland contains: (T/F)
a) The facial nerve (T)
b) The external carotid artery (T)
c) The superficial temporal artery (F)
d) The retromandibular vein (T)

17. The temporal fossa (T/F)
a) Is entirely located over the temporal bone (F-the temporal fossa is located over the frontal, the sphenoid, the temporal, the parietal and the occipital bones)
b) Has the zygomatic arch inferior to it (T-the zygomatic arch and the wing of the sphenoid form the inferior border of the temporal fossa)
c) Contains the superficial temporal artery (T)
d) Contains the deep temporal nerves (T-these branch off the mandibular division of the trigeminal nerve)

The temporal fossa is located superficially on the side of the head and contains numerous structures that can be damaged following injury to the side of the head

18. The nasal cavity: (T/F)
a) Has 3 turbinates on each side (T-these increase the surface area of the nasal cavity, allowing air to be warmed and to provide an increased surface area of cilia to filter air)
b) Is innervated by the trigeminal nerve (T)
c) Has its blood supply from the maxillary artery only (F-the blood supply is from the facial, maxillary and ethmoidal arteries)
d) The nasolacrimal duct drains into the middle meatus (F-the nasolacrimal duct drains into the inferior meatus)

19. The subclavian vein: (T/F)
a) Is the continuation of the axillary vein (T)
b) Commences at the medial border of the clavicle (F-the subclavian vein commences at the outer border of the 1st rib)
c) Contributes to the formation of the brachiocephalic vein (T-the subclavian and internal jugular veins unite to form the brachiocephalic vein)
d) Has the thoracic duct draining into it on the right side (F-the left subclavian vein has the thoracic duct draining into it at its junction with the internal jugular vein)

20. Regarding the facial nerve: (T/F)
a) It supplies taste fibres to the posterior third of the tongue (F-the facial nerve, via the chorda tympani, supplies the submandibular and sublingual salivary glands, as well as taste fibres to the anterior two-thirds of the tongue. The glossopharyngeal nerve supplies taste fibres to the posterior third of the tongue)
b) It supplies all the muscles of facial expression (T-the trigeminal nerve supplies the muscles of mastication (masseter, temporalis, pterygoids), but none of these can be considered muscles of facial expression. The facial nerve controls all the muscles of facial expression)

c) It can be tested using the corneal reflex (T-the corneal reflex tests both the trigeminal and facial nerves, which supply the afferent and efferent arcs of the reflex respectively. If the patient can feel the cotton wool used for testing, but does not blink, a facial nerve palsy is present. If the patient cannot feel the cotton wool, then a trigeminal nerve palsy is present)
d) It can be damaged by wounds in the pre-auricular area (T-wounds anterior to the external auditory meatus can be associated with facial nerve damage, due to the relatively superficial position of the facial nerve within the parotid gland in this area)

21. Orbicularis oculi: (T/F)
a) Is supplied only by the temporal branch of the facial nerve (F-orbicularis oculiis is supplied by the temporal and zygomatic branches of the facial nerve)
b) Closes the eyelids (T-the palpebral and orbital components of the orbicularis oculi close the eyelid)
c) Empties the lacrimal sac (T-the lacrimal component of orbicularis oculi draws the eyelids and the ends of the lacrimal canals medially and compresses them against the globe. This places them in the most favourable situation for receiving tears from the lacrimal sac, which it also compresses)
d) Is not used in the corneal reflex (F-the action of blinking when the cornea is stimulated is carried out by orbicularis oculi)

22. The pterygoid venous plexus: (T/F)
a) Communicates with the cavernous sinus (T-by venous branches through the foramen venosum, foramen ovale, and foramen lacerum)
b) Is situated between the temporalis and medial pterygoid (F-it is situated between the temporalis and the lateral pterygoid)

c) Can be damaged during dental procedures (T-posterior superior alveolar nerve blocks, which are used to anaesthetise multiple molar teeth, can cause haematomas of the pterygoid venous plexus if not accurately performed)
d) Communicates with the ophthalmic vein (T-through the inferior orbital fissure)

23. Regarding the opthalmic division of the trigeminal nerve: (T/F)
a) The opthalmic nerve is a mixed motor and sensory nerve (F-the opthalmic nerve is entirely sensory)
b) The infratrochlear nerve supples the skin of the eyelids (T)
c) The frontal nerve supplies the skin at the tip of the nose (F-the external nasal nerve, a branch of the nasociliary nerve, supplies the skin at the tip of the nose)
d) The frontal nerve supplies the skin of the forehead and scalp (T-this is via the supraorbital and supratrochlear nerves. These nerves can be blocked using local anaesthetic to facilitate wound management on the forehead and scalp)

24. Buccinator: (T/F)
a) Arises entirely from the maxilla and mandible (F-buccinator arises from the maxilla, the mandible and from the pterygomandibular ligament)
b) Is supplied by the mandibular branch of the facial nerve (F-buccinator is supplied by the buccal branch of the facial nerve)
c) Pulls the angle of the mouth forwards (F-buccinator pulls the angle of the mouth backwards, as in smiling)
d) Inserts into the orbicularis oris (T-the fibres of buccinator insert into orbicularis oris as well as into the lips)

25. Regarding the branches of the external carotid artery: (T/F)
a) The facial artery supplies the tonsils (T)
b) Injury to the middle meningeal artery classically results in a subdural haematoma (F-significant injury to the middle meningeal artery results in an extradural haematoma)
c) The maxillary artery is given off from the external carotid artery within the parotid gland (T)
d) Branches of the occipital artery supplies the pinna (F-the anterior and posterior auricular arteries, branches of the superficial temporal and external carotid arteries respectively, supply the external auditory meatus and pinna)

26. Regarding the submandibular lymph nodes: (T/F)
a) They receive lymph from the entire upper and lower lips (F-the submental nodes receive lymph from the central portion of the lower lip, the submandibular nodes drain lymph from the rest of the lips)
b) They receive lymph from the entire tongue (F-the submental nodes receive lymph from the tip of the tongue, the submandibular nodes drain lymph from the rest of the tongue)
c) They receive lymph from the front of the scalp (T)
d) They receive lymph from the facial sinuses (T-the submandibular lymph nodes receive lymph from the frontal, ethmoid and maxillary sinuses)

27. Occipitofrontalis: (T/F)
a) Has 2 bellies (T-the occipital and frontal bellies)
b) Is innervated by the facial nerve (T)
c) Originates in part from the frontal bone (F-occipitofrontalis has 2 points of origin; from the occipital bone and from the skin/fascia of the eyebrow)
d) Raises the eyebrow (T-occipitofrontalis also moves the

scalp)

28. Regarding the blood supply to the scalp: (T/F)
a) It is derived entirely from the external carotid artery (F-the blood supply to the scalp is derived from the internal and external carotid arteries)
b) The posterior auricular artery supplies the pinna (T)
c) The supraorbital artery does not supply the scalp (F-the supraorbital artery passes through the supraorbital foramen and supplies the muscles and the pericranium of the forehead. It anastomoses with the supratrochlear artery and the frontal branch of the superficial temporal artery. This is an example of the complex series of anastomoses between the internal and external carotid arteries that supply the scalp)
d) The superficial temporal artery is impalpable (F-the superficial temporal artery is easily palpated anterior to the tragus)

29. Regarding the veins of the cranium and brain: (T/F)
a) They have no valves (T)
b) They have thick walls (F-the veins of the brain have thin walls, making them vulnerable to injury)
c) They drain to the venous sinuses (T)
d) The diploic veins are situated in the cranial bones (T-the diploic veins are situated within the skull itself and drain into the venous sinuses)

30. Regarding the temporal bone: (T/F)
a) It has 5 bony components (T-the temporal bone has 5 components; the squamous (which includes the zygomatic process), the petrous, tympanic, the mastoid process and the styloid process)
b) The temporal line is located on the temporal bone (F-the temporal line is located on the parietal bone. It gives attachment to the temporal fascia and indicates the upper

limit of the temporalis)
c) It has the ethmoid bone immediately anterior to it (F-the sphenoid is immediately anterior to the temporal bone)
d) It forms part of the temporal fossa (T)

31. Masseter: (T/F)
a) Originates from the zygomatic arch (T)
b) Is supplied by the facial nerve (F-it is supplied by the mandibular branch of the trigeminal nerve)
c) Assists in chewing (T-masseter closes the mouth by raising the mandible)
d) Inserts into the body of the mandible (F-it inserts into the mandibular ramus and the coronoid process)

32. Regarding the parotid gland: (T/F)
a) It has 2 lobes (T-the superficial and deep lobes)
b) It is innervated by the facial nerve (F-the glossopharyngeal nerve supplies the parotid gland. The facial nerve traverses the parotid gland, but does not supply it)
c) Its duct passes between the masseter and buccinator (F-the parotid duct traverses the masseter and then travels through the buccinator fibres to open in the mouth opposite the 2nd upper molar)
d) It is the smallest salivary gland (F-it is the largest salivary gland)

33. Regarding the maxillary division of the trigeminal nerve: (T/F)
a) The maxillary nerve is a mixed motor and sensory nerve (F-the maxillary nerve is entirely sensory)
b) It supplies the skin on the side of the nose (T-the infraorbital nerve supplies the skin of the anterior face and side of the nose. It can be blocked using local anaesthetic to facilitate wound management on the face)

c) The anterior superior alveolar nerve supplies the upper pre-molar teeth (F-the anterior superior alveolar nerve supplies the upper canines and incisors. The middle superior alveolar nerve supplies the upper pre-molar teeth)
d) The superior alveolar nerves supply the maxillary sinus (T-as well as the upper teeth, the alveolar nerves supply the maxillary sinus)

34. The infratemporal fossa: (T/F)
a) Is situated medial to the zygomatic arch (T-the infratemporal fossa lies inferior and medial to the zygomatic arch)
b) Contains the mandibular and maxillary nerves (T)
c) Has the foramen rotundum within its borders (F-it has the foramen ovale and foranum spinosum within its borders. The foramen ovale transmits the mandibular division of the trigeminal nerve and the lesser petrosal nerve. The foramen spinosum transmits the middle meningeal artery)
d) Has the medial pterygoid as its floor (T)

35. The maxillary artery: (T/F)
a) Is a branch of the internal carotid artery (F-it is a branch of the external carotid artery)
b) Gives off the middle meningeal artery (T)
c) Supplies the pterygoids (T-the maxillary artery supplies the muscles of mastication)
d) Supplies the palate (T-via the palatine arteries)

36. Regarding the mandibular nerve: (T/F)
a) It is a division of the facial nerve (F-it is a division of the trigeminal nerve)
b) It is transmitted via the foramen ovale (T)
c) It is entirely sensory (F-it is a mixed motor and sensory nerve)

d) It has 3 divisions (F-it has 2 divisions, anterior and posterior)

37. Temporalis: (T/F)
a) Originates from the temporal fossa (T)
b) Inserts into the mandible (T-specifically, temporalis inserts into the coronoid process of the mandible)
c) Is innervated by the deep temporal nerves (F-temporalis is innervated by the mandibular division of the trigeminal nerve)
d) Retracts the mandible (T-temporalis retracts and elevates the mandible)

38. Regarding the branches of the trigeminal nerve: (T/F)
a) The auriculotemporal nerve supplies the external auditory meatus (T)
b) The lingual nerve transmits taste fibres from the anterior two-thirds of the tongue (F-the lingual nerve transmits somatic sensory information, e.g. pain and temperature from the anterior two-thirds of the tongue)
c) The inferior alveolar nerve supplies the skin of the chin (T-the inferior alveolar nerve also supplies the lower teeth)
d) The buccal nerve supplies buccinator (F-the buccal nerve supplies the skin of the cheek. The facial nerve supplies buccinator)

39. The hypoglossal nerve: (T/F)
a) Is a mixed motor and sensory nerve (F-it is entirely motor)
b) Descends through the skull via the jugular foramen (F-it descends through the skull via the hypoglossal canal)
c) Supplies all the muscles of the tongue (F-the hypoglossal nerve supplies all the muscles of the tongue except palatoglossus, which is innervated by the pharyngeal plexus)

d) Travels within the carotid sheath (T-the hypoglossal nerve travels through the superior portion of the carotid sheath)

40. The following are components of the roof of the nose: (T/F)
a) The body of the sphenoid (T)
b) The nasal septum (F)
c) The cribriform plate (T)
d) The frontal bone (T)

The roof of the nose is made up of the body of the sphenoid, the nasal bone, the cribriform plate and the frontal bone

41. Regarding the mandibular division of the trigeminal nerve: (T/F)
a) The mandibular nerve is a mixed motor and sensory nerve (T-the masseter, temporalis and pterygoids are all supplied by branches of the mandibular nerve, as are the mylohyoid and anterior belly of digastric)
b) It supplies the anterior two-thirds of the tongue (T-the lingual nerve and the chorda tympani supply the anterior two-thirds of the tongue. Importantly, the lingual nerve transmits somatic sensory information e.g. pain and temporature, whilst the chordae tympani transmits taste)
c) It supplies the submandibular salivary glands (T-the chordae tympani and the lingual nerve jointly supply the submandibular salivary glands)
d) It supplies the parotid salivary gland (T-the auriculotemporal nerve supplies the parotid salivary gland along with the glossopharyngeal nerve, via the lesser petrosal nerve)

42. The external carotid artery: (T/F)
a) Begins at the level of the cricoid cartilage (F-the external carotid artery branches from the common

carotid artery at the level of the upper border of the thyroid cartilage)
b) Gives off the inferior thyroid artery (F-the inferior thyroid artery is a branch of the thyrocervical trunk)
c) Runs superficial to platysma (F-the external carotid artery is deep to platysma)
d) Gives off the lingual artery (T)

43. The arteries that anastomose in Little's area include: (T/F)
a) The posterior ethmoidal artery (F)
b) The sphenopalatine artery (T)
c) The greater palatine artery (T)
d) The nasal artery (F)

The arteries that anastomose in Little's area are the anterior ethmoidal, the sphenopalatine, the greater palatine and the superior labial arteries

44. Regarding the teeth: (T/F)
a) There are 34 permanent teeth (F-there are 32 permanent teeth)
b) The permanent incisors erupt at age 7 to 8 years (T)
c) The deciduous molars erupt at age 6 to 8 months (F-the deciduous molars erupt at age 10 to 24 months)
d) The permanent canines erupt at age 11 to 12 years (T)

45. Regarding the adenoids and tonsils: (T/F)
a) The adenoids are situated in the oropharynx (F-the adenoids are situated in the nasopharynx)
b) The palatine tonsils are supplied by the lingual artery (T)
c) Peritonsillar abscesses are usually bilateral (F-they are usually unilateral)
d) The tonsils drain to the superficial cervical chain of lymph nodes (F-the tonsils drain to the jugulodigastric

nodes)

46. Regarding the laryngeal cartilages: (T/F)
a) The cricoid cartilage is the largest of the laryngeal cartilages (F-the thyroid cartilage is the largest of the laryngeal cartilages)
b) The cricoid cartilage lies superior to the thyroid cartilage (F-the cricoid cartilage lies inferior to the thyroid cartilage)
c) The arytenoid cartilages have vocal processes (T-each aretynoid cartilage has a muscular and vocal process, an apex and a base)
d) The corniculate cartilages are cone shaped (T)

47. Regarding the larynx: (T/F)
a) The internal laryngeal nerve runs through the thyrohyoid membrane (T-the internal laryngeal nerve is the internal branch of the superior laryngeal nerve. It pierces the thyrohyoid membrane and then is distributed to the mucous membrane of the larynx)
b) The quadrangular membrane lies between the epiglottis and the thryoid cartilage (F-the quadrangular membrane lies between the epiglottis and the arytenoid cartilages)
c) The digastric muscle attaches to the hyoid bone (T-both the anterior and posterior bellies of digastric attach to the hyoid)
d) The epiglottis is attached to the cricoid cartilage (F-the epiglottis is attached to the thyroid cartilage)

48. Regarding the auditory ossicles: (T/F)
a) The malleus is the largest of the ossicles (T)
b) The incus is attached to the oval window (F-the stapes is attached to the oval window by the annular ligament)
c) The malleus is attached to the tympanic membrane (T)
d) The tensor tympani muscle enhances transmission of sound from the tympanic membrane to the ossicles (F-the

tensor tympani reduces the vibrations of the tympanic membrane)

49. Regarding the recurrent laryngeal nerve: (T/F)
a) Unilateral recurrent laryngeal nerve damage has no discernible clinical effect (F unilateral damage to the recurrent laryngeal nerve results in a hoarse voice)
b) Bilateral recurrent laryngeal nerve damage can result in airway compromise (T-if bilateral recurrent laryngeal nerve damage occurs, the vocal cords become paralysed, potentially leading to airway compromise)
c) It may be damaged in thyroid surgery: (T-the recurrent laryngeal nerve runs posteromedially to the thyroid and must be clearly identified during thyroid surgery to avoid damage)
d) The right recurrent laryngeal nerve is longer than the left: (F-the left recurrent laryngeal nerve is longer than the right)

50. Regarding the bony margins of the orbit: (T/F)
a) The roof of the orbit is formed by the frontal bone only (F-the roof of the orbit is formed by the frontal bone and the lesser wing of the sphenoid)
b) The lateral wall of the orbit is formed by the zygoma only (F-the lateral wall of the orbit is formed by the zygoma and the greater wing of the sphenoid)
c) The floor of the orbit is formed by the maxilla only (T-the orbital plate of the maxilla separates the orbit from the maxillary sinus)
d) The nasolacrimal canal is on the roof of the orbit (F-the nasolacrimal canal is on the medial wall of the orbit)

51. Regarding the eyelids: (T/F)
a) They contain a fibrous septum (T-the orbital septum is a fibrous framework within the eyelids)
b) The palpebral ligaments attach the tarsal plates to the

orbit (T-the lateral and medial palpebral ligaments attach the tarsal plates to the orbital margins)
c) The orbicularis oculi opens the eyes (F-orbicularis oculi closes the eyes)
d) The levator palpebrae superioris opens the eye (T-it does this by raising the upper eyelid)

52. The accessory nerve: (T/F)
a) Is a mixed motor and sensory nerve (F-it is entirely motor)
b) Descends through the skull via the jugular foramen (T)
c) Innervates the pharynx (T-the cranial root of the accessory nerve contributes to the innervation of the pharynx via the pharyngeal plexus)
d) Supplies the sternocleidomastoid (T-it also supplies the trapezius)

53. Regarding the contents of the eye: (T/F)
a) The aqueous humor fills both the anterior and posterior chambers (T)
b) The vitreous body is a pigmented gel (F-the vitreous body is a transparent gel)
c) The lens is a bi-concave structure (F-the lens is a bi-convex structure)
d) The lens is attached to the ciliary body (T-the lens is attached to the ciliary body by the suspensory ligament)

54. Regarding the lacrimal apparatus: (T/F)
a) The lacrimal gland is supplied by the facial nerve (T)
b) Tears enter the lacrimal sac via the canaliculi (T-the canaliculi open into the lacrimal sac)
c) The lacrimal gland lies on the medial wall of the orbit (F-the lacrimal gland lies in the supero-anterior aspect of the orbit)
d) The nasolacrimal duct enters the nose in the superior meatus (F-the nasolacrimal duct enters the nose in the

inferior meatus)

55. Regarding the extrinsic orbital muscles: (T/F)
a) Superior rectus raises the eye upwards (T)
b) Lateral rectus rotates the eye to look outwards (T)
c) Superior oblique is innervated by the abducent nerve (F-superior oblique is innervated by the trochlear nerve)
d) Inferior oblique is innervated by the oculomotor nerve (T)

56. Regarding the auditory tube: (T/F)
a) The auditory tube links the middle ear to the oropharynx (F-the auditory tube links the middle ear to the nasopharynx)
b) The mastoid antrum connects to the inner ear (F-the mastoid antrum, which lies in the petrous temporal bone, connects to the middle ear)
c) The mastoid air cells are continuous with the middle ear (T)
d) Mastoiditis is commonly related to otitis media (T-otitis media is one of the commonest causes of mastoiditis)

57. The optic nerve: (T/F)
a) Enters the cranium through the ethmoid bone (F-the optic nerve enters the cranium via the optic canal in the sphenoid bone)
b) Crosses the midline (T-fibres from the medial half of the retina cross the midline in the optic chiasm. Fibres from the lateral half of the retina do not cross the midline)
c) Can be inflamed in patients with multiple sclerosis (T-optic neuritis is often associated with multiple sclerosis)
d) Is myelinated (T)

58. The temporomandibular joint: (T/F)
a) Is a synovial joint (T)

b) Is the articulation between the temporal bone and mandibular head (T-the mandibular joint is the articulation between the temporal bone, the mandibular fossa and the head of the mandible)
c) Has no capsule (F-the temporomandibular joint has a joint capsule)
d) Is rarely dislocated in the absence of direct trauma (F-dislocations of the temporomandibular joint are frequently atraumatic. Yawning is a common cause)

59. Regarding the brain: (T/F)
a) The central sulcus separates the frontal lobe from the occipital lobe (F-the central sulcus separates the frontal lobe from the parietal lobe)
b) The lateral sulcus separates the parietal lobe from the temporal lobe (F-the lateral sulcus separates the frontal lobe from the temporal lobe)
c) The occipital lobe is the smallest lobe (T)
d) The corpus callosum connects the right and left sides of the brain (T-the corpus callosum connects the left and right hemispheres and facilitates communication between them)

60. Regarding damaged areas of the brain: (T/F)
a) Damage to Broca's area causes difficulty with speaking (T-damage to Broca's area, located at the inferior frontal gyrus, causes various speech disorders including aphasia and loss of language comprehension)
b) Damage to Wernicke's area causes difficulty with limb coordination (F-Wernicke's area, located at the posterior aspect of the superior temporal gyrus, has a role in speech processing and damage to it causes speech difficulties)
c) Damage to the occipital lobe causes hearing problems (F-the primary auditory cortex is in the temporal lobe. The frontal and parietal lobes also have roles in sound processing, but not the occipital lobe)

d) Posterior cerebral artery occlusion causes visual symptoms (T-the posterior cerebral artery supplies the occipital lobe and hence the visual cortex. Occlusion of the posterior cerebral artery can cause visual field deficits and cortical blindness)

61. The optic nerve: (T/F)
a) Arises within the retina (T-the optic nerve arises from axons in the retinal ganglion cells)
b) Enters the cranium in the anterior cranial fossa (F-the optic nerve enters the cranium in the middle cranial fossa)
c) All its fibres cross the midline (F-fibres from the medial half of the retina cross the midline. Fibres from the lateral half of the retina pass ipsilaterally in the optic tract)
d) All the nerve fibres synapse within the lateral geniculate body (F-most of the nerve fibres synapse within the lateral geniculate body. Some fibres terminate in the pretectal nucleus and superior colliculus of the mid-brain, these fibres are involved in light reflexes)

62. The internal carotid artery: (T/F)
a) Enters the cranium via the jugular foramen (F-the internal carotid artery enters the cranium by passing in the carotid canal within the petrous temporal bone, then exiting between the lingula and petrosal process of the sphenoid)
b) Gives off the opthalmic artery (T)
c) Gives off the occipital artery (F-the occipital artery is a branch of the external carotid artery)
d) Gives off the posterior communicating artery (T)

63. The following arteries are components of the circle of Willis: (T/F)
a) Anterior cerebral artery (T)

b) Middle cerebral artery (F-the middle cerebral artery is a terminal branch of the internal carotid. Some anatomists include it as part of the circle of Willis, however, the general consensus is that it is not part of the circle of Willis)
c) Posterior communicating artery (T)
d) Basilar artery (T)

The circle of Willis *is a site of anastomosis between the internal carotid and vertebral arteries. It is made up of the following arteries:*
Anterior communicating artery
Anterior cerebral artery
Posterior communicating artery
Posterior cerebral artery
Basilar artery

64. The vagus nerve: (T/F)
a) Arises from the brain stem (T-the vagus nerve arises from the medulla oblongata)
b) Leaves the skull through the foramen lacerum (F-the vagus nerve leaves the skull through the jugular foramen)
c) Travels in the carotid sheath (T)
d) Passes through the diaphragm through the aortic opening (F-the vagus nerve passes through the diaphragm through the oesophageal opening)

65. Regarding the spinothalamic tracts: (T/F)
a) They transmit pain and temperature (T)
b) The fibres decussate in the brain stem (F-the fibres decussate in the spinal cord)
c) Are situated anteriorly in the spinal cord (F-the spinothalamic tracts are situated laterally in the spinal cord)

d) Only utilise C fibres to convey nociception (F-the spinothalamic tracts utilise A and C fibres to transmit pain)

66. The following are correctly paired clinical findings and GCS scores: (T/F)
a) Eyes opening to pain - E2 (T)
b) Incomprehensible sounds - V3 (F-incomprehensible sounds corresponds to a verbal response score of V2)
c) Abnormal flexion - M3 (T)
d) Localises pain - M4 (F-localising to pain corresponds to a motor score of M5)

67. Signs of carotid artery dissection include: (T/F)
a) Horner's syndrome (T)
b) Headache (T)
c) Hemiparesis (T)
d) Amaurosis fugax (T)

Vertebral artery dissection can result in numerous symptoms. These can be very non-specific and result from arterial occlusion at the site of the dissection, and/or the effects of emboli that originate from the dissection

68. Regarding the external auditory meatus: (T/F)
a) The pinna is a cartilaginous structure (T)
b) The ear canal is approximately 3cm in length (T)
c) Its blood supply is from the facial artery (F-the anterior and posterior auricular arteries, branches of the superficial temporal and external carotid arteries respectively, supply the external auditory meatus)
d) The external surface of the tympanic membrane is supplied solely by the trigeminal nerve (F-the external surface of the tympanic membrane is supplied by the trigeminal nerve and the vagus nerve)

69. Within the eyeball: (T/F)
a) The sclera lies anterior to the cornea (F-the cornea lies anterior to the sclera)
b) The sclera never connects with the cornea (F-the sclera is connected to the cornea at the corneoscleral junction, known as the limbus)
c) The choroid has a pigmented layer (T-the outer layer of the choroid is pigmented)
d) The ciliary muscles change the shape of the lens (T-supplied by the oculomotor nerve, the ciliary muscles cause the lens to alter shape)

70. The middle cerebral artery: (T/F)
a) Is the largest branch of the internal carotid artery (T)
b) Supplies the entire motor cortex (F-the middle cerebral artery supplies the entire motor cortex except the area which supplies the legs)
c) When occluded, causes a contralateral hemiplegia affecting the face (T)
d) When occluded, causes a sensory loss of the ipsilateral sensory loss affecting the arm (F-an occlusion of the middle cerebral artery causes a contralateral hemiplegia and hemiparesis)

71. The following movements of the jaw are correctly associated with the named muscles: (T/F)
a) Jaw protrusion - medial pterygoid (F-jaw protrusion is enacted by the lateral pterygoid)
b) Jaw retraction - temporalis (T)
c) Mouth opening - digastric (T-mandibular elevation is also enacted by the geniohyoid and mylohyoid muscles)
d) Mouth closing - lateral pterygoid (F-mandibular depression is enacted by the medial pterygoid as well as temporalis and masseter)

72. The sternocleidomastoid muscle: (T/F)
a) Is supplied by the accessory nerve (T-the sternocleidomastoid is also supplied by the C2 and C3 spinal nerves via the accessory nerve)
b) Has the external jugular vein deep to it (F-the external jugular vein lies superficial to the sternocleidomastoid. This makes it a useful site for intravenous cannulation in emergencies)
c) Divides the neck into anterior and posterior triangles (T)
d) Has platysma superficial to it (T)

73. The internal jugular vein: (T/F)
a) Commences as the continuation of the sagittal sinus (F-the internal jugular vein commences as the continuation of the sigmoid venous sinus)
b) Runs in the carotid sheath (T)
c) Contributes to the formation of the brachiocephalic vein (T-the internal jugular vein joins the subclavian vein the form the brachiocephalic vein)
d) Receives the venous drainage of the entire thyroid gland (F-the superior and middle thyroid veins drain into the internal jugular vein. The inferior thyroid vein drains into the left brachiocephalic vein)

74. The posterior triangle of the neck: (T/F)
a) Is bounded anteriorly by the sternocleidomastoid (T-the posterior border of the sternocleidomastoid is the anterior border of the posterior triangle)
b) Is bounded posteriorly by the trapezius (T-the anterior border of the trapezius is the posterior border of the posterior triangle)
c) Has the inferior belly of omohyoid as its inferior border (F-the clavicle is the inferior border of the posterior triangle)
d) Has the insertion of the sternocleidomastoid as its apex

(F-the apex of the posterior triangle is the union of sternocleidomastoid and trapezius at the occipital bone)

75. Regarding the thyroid gland: (T/F)
a) It has the carotid sheath running anterolaterally to it (F-the carotid sheath runs posterolaterally to the thyroid)
b) It has the infrahyoid muscles posterior to it (F-the infrahyoid muscles run anterolaterally to the thyroid, as does the anterior border of sternocleidomastoid)
c) Its isthmus lies in the midline anterior to the 2nd to 4th tracheal rings (T)
d) It is surrounded by a fascial sheath (T-this pre-tracheal fascia attaches the thyroid to the trachea and larynx)

76. The phrenic nerve: (T/F)
a) Arises from the 3rd to 5th cervical nerves (T-the phrenic nerve is formed from the anterior rami of the 3rd to 5th cervical nodes)
b) Descends medial to the vagus nerve within the thorax (F-the phrenic nerve decends laterally to the vagus nerve in the thorax)
c) Runs medially to the roots of each lung (F-the phrenic nerve runs in front of the root of the lung on both sides)
d) Passes anteriorly to the scalenus anterior (T)

77. The external jugular vein: (T/F)
a) Runs deep to the sternocleidomastoid (F-the external jugular vein runs superficially to the sternocleidomastoid. This allows it to be used for intravenous cannulation in emergency situations)
b) Is formed by the union of the posterior auricular and the temporal vein (F-the external jugular vein is formed by the union of the posterior auricular and the posterior retromandibular vein)
c) Drains into the subclavian vein (T-the external jugular vein drains into the subclavian vein behind the clavicle)

d) Runs deep to platysma (T)

78. Regarding the extrinsic orbital muscles: (T/F)
a) Superior oblique rotates the eye to look upwards and outwards (F-superior oblique rotates the eye to look downwards and outwards)
b) Medial rectus rotates the eye to look inwards (T)
c) Inferior rectus can be damaged in orbital floor fractures (T-the inferior rectus can be injured in an orbital floor fracture. This leads to diplopia and an inability to look upwards and inwards)
d) Lateral rectus is innervated by the oculomotor nerve (F-lateral rectus is innervated by the abducent nerve)

79. Regarding the ventricular system of the brain: (T/F)
a) CSF is produced in all parts of the ventricular system (F-CSF is produced in the choroid plexus, which is found in all parts of the ventricular system except the cerebral aquaduct, and the anterior and posterior horns of the lateral ventricles)
b) CSF travels between the lateral ventricles and the 3rd ventricle via the foramen of Luschka (F-CSF travels between the lateral ventricles and the third ventricle via the foramen of Monro)
c) CSF travels between the 3rd and 4th ventricles via the cerebral aquaduct (T)
d) CSF drains into the venous system via the superior sagittal sinus (T-CSF is absobed into the venous system via the arachnoid vill in the superior sagittal sinus)

80. Orbicularis oris: (T/F)
a) Is supplied by the buccal branch of the facial nerve (T)
b) Arises entirely from the maxilla and mandible (F- orbicularis oris rises from the maxilla, the mandible, the skin of the lips and the buccinator)
c) Closes the mouth (T-orbicularis oris closes the mouth and puckers the lips)
d) Surrounds the entire mouth (T)

SPINE ANSWERS

1. The following vertebral groups have the correct number of vertebrae: (T/F)
a) Thoracic - 12 (T)
b) Lumbar - 5 (T)
c) Sacral - 3 (F-there are 5 sacral vertebrae, which are fused to form the sacrum)
d) Coccygeal - 3 (F-there are 4 coccygeal vertebrae. The lower 3 are often fused)

2. Regarding examination findings in spinal injury: (T/F)
a) A patient with grade 2 motor function will be able to lift a limb against gravity (F-grade 2 motor function means the patient can move a limb with gravity eliminated, grade 3 motor function means a patient will be able to lift a limb against gravity)
b) An intact bulbocavernosus reflex means that sacral sparing is conclusively present (F-an intact bulbocavernosus reflex shows that the S1 to 3 nerves are intact, an intact anal cutaneous reflex (S4 and 5) in addition to an intact bulbocavernosus reflex means that sacral sparing is present)
c) A patient with grade 1 motor function will have visible muscular contractions (T)
d) Lack of spinal tenderness means that the vertebral bodies are intact (F-it is possible to have significant vertebral injuries in the absence of spinal tenderness. Spinal percussion may elicit signs of vertebral injury)

3. Each vertebrae contains: (T/F)
a) 4 pedicles (F-there are 2 pedicles on each vertebrae. These form the posterior vertebral arch)
b) 1 spinous process (T)
c) 2 transverse process (T)
d) 2 articular processes (F-there are 4 articular processes

on each vertebrae)

4. Regarding the intervertebral discs: (T/F)
a) The intervertebral discs are thicker in the thoracic region than in the cervical region (F-the discs are thickest in the cervical and lumbar regions)
b) The anulus fibrosus attaches to the anterior longitudinal ligament only (F-the anulus fibrosus attaches to the anterior and posterior longitudinal ligaments)
c) The nucleus pulposus becomes dehydrated with age (T-the nucleus pulposus is comprised of gelatinous material. The water content of this gelatinous material decreases with age and is replaced by fibrocartilage)
d) There are no discs in the sacrum (T-there are no discs in the sacrum or coccyx)

5. Regarding the spinal ligaments: (T/F)
a) The ligamentum flavum connects the spinous processes of adjacent vertebrae (F-the ligamentum flavum connects the laminae of adjacent vertebrae)
b) The supraspinous ligament connects the spinous process of one vertebrae to the transverse process of the adjacent vertebrae (F-the supraspinous ligament connects the spinous processes of adjacent vertebrae to each other)
c) The interspinous ligament connects the spinous process of one vertebrae to the spinous process of the adjacent vertebrae (T)
d) The ligamentum nuchae is only present in the cervical vertebrae (T)

6. Regarding the atlanto-occipital joints: (T/F)
a) The atlanto-occipital joints are not synovial joints (F-the atlanto-occipital joints are synovial joints)
b) The atlanto-occipital joints have capsules (T)
c) The anterior altlanto-occipital membrane connects the arch of the atlas to the foramen magnum (T-specifically,

the anterior altlanto-occipital membrane connects the anterior arch of the atlas to the anterior edge of the foramen magnum)
d) Rotation is possible at the atlanto-occipital joints (F- rotation is not possible at the atlanto-occipital joints, but flexion, extension and lateral flexion are)

7. Anterior cord syndrome: (T/F)
a) Causes a loss of proprioception and light touch (F- proprioception and light touch are functions of the posterior column, they are preserved in anterior cord syndrome)
b) Causes complete paralysis below the injury (T)
c) Causes loss of pain below the injury (T)
d) Has an excellent prognosis (F-the prognosis for anterior cord syndrome is poor)

8. The following structures are clearly visible on a correctly positioned odontoid peg radiograph: (T/F)
a) Lateral mass of C1 (T)
b) Body of C2 (T)
c) Dens (T-the dens is the odontoid peg. It is clearly visible on a peg radiograph)
d) Spinous process of C1 (F-the first cervical vertebrae has a rudimentary posterior tubercle to which the ligamentum nuchae attaches, but no spinous process)

9. The first cervical vertebrae: (T/F)
a) Has no spinous process (T-C1 has a rudimentary posterior tubercle, to which the ligamentum nuchae attaches, but no spinous process)
b) Has a vertebral body (F-C1 is a ring shaped structure and has no vertebral body)
c) Has no transverse processes (F-C1 has transverse processes on both sides)
d) Articulates with the occipital condyles (T)

10. Regarding the atlantoaxial joints: (T/F)
a) The atlantoaxial joints are synovial joints (T)
b) The atlantoaxial joints have capsules (T)
c) There are 2 atlantoaxial joints (F-there are 3 atlantoaxial joints, one between the odontoid process and the anterior arch of the atlas, and two between the lateral masses)
d) There is no rotation at the atlantoaxial joints (F-the atlantoaxial joints allow rotation of the head)

11. Regarding the layers of the meninges: (T/F)
a) The dura mater surrouding the spine is continuous with the dura of the brain (T)
b) The arachnoid mater is semi-permeable to fluid (F-the arachnoid mater is impermeable to fluid)
c) The sub-arachnoid space lies between the pia and the arachnoid mater (T)
d) The dura does not envelop the spinal nerve roots (F-the dura gives off sheaths to the spinal nerve roots)

12. Brown-Sequard syndrome: (T/F)
a) Is the result of complete spinal cord transection (F-Brown-Sequard syndrome occurs after hemisection of the spinal cord)
b) Is more common in penetrating injuries than blunt injuries (T)
c) Causes ipsilateral loss of pain and temperature sensation (F-contralateral loss of pain and temperature is seen in Brown-Sequard syndrome due to the decussation of the fibres within the spinothalamic tracts being within the spinal cord)
d) Causes ipsilateral loss of power and sensation (T)

13. Regarding the ligaments of the atlantoaxial joints: (T/F)
a) The vertical part of the cruciate ligament connects the

axis to the foramen magnum (T-specifically, the vertical part of the cruciate ligament connects the body of the axis to the anterior edge of the foramen magnum)
b) The transverse part of the cruciate ligament connects the odontoid process to the atlas (T-specifically, the transverse part of the cruciate ligament connects the odontoid process to the anterior arch of the atlas)
c) The alar ligaments connect the odontoid process to the transverse process of the atlas (F-the alar ligaments connect the odontoid process to the occipital condyles)
d) The apical ligament connects the odontoid process to the foramen magnum (T-specifically, the apical ligament connects the odontoid process to the anterior edge of the foramen magnum)

14. The spinal cord: (T/F)
a) In adults, ends at the lower border of the L1 vertebrae (T)
b) Is surrounded by 4 meningeal layers (F-the spinal cord is surrounded by 3 meningeal layers - the dura mater, the arachnoid mater and the pia mater)
c) Is continuous with the medulla oblongata (T)
d) Has 4 fissures (F-the spinal cord has 2 fissures - the anterior and posterior median fissures, also known as the posterior median sulcus)

15. Regarding the spinal nerves: (T/F)
a) There are 31 pairs of spinal nerves (T-these are attached to the cord by the anterior and posterior nerve roots)
b) The anterior nerve roots are motor (T-the anterior nerve roots are motor, the posterior nerve roots are sensory)
c) The spinal nerves unite to form the anterior and posterior rami before they pass through the intervertebral foramen (F-the spinal nerve form the

anterior and posterior rami after passing through the intervertebral foramen)
d) The anterior rami only contain sensory fibres (F-the anterior rami contain sensory and motor fibres)

16. During a correctly performed lumbar puncture, the needle passes through the: (T/F)
a) Supraspinous ligament (T)
b) Ligamentum flavum (T)
c) Ligamentum nuchae (F-the ligamentum nuchae is only present in the cervical spine)
d) Erector spinae (F-the erector spinae group of muscles are situated on the sides of the spinous processes. As they are not in the midline, they should not be pierced during a lumbar puncture)

17. Viewed from the side, the following descriptions of the spine are correct: (T/F)
a) The cervical spine is posteriorly concave (T)
b) The lumbar spine is posteriorly concave (T)
c) A pregnant woman will have a decreased lumbar posterior concavity (F-due to the weight and size of the foetus, the lumbar spine has a increased posterior lumbar concavity- a lordosis)
d) An older person will develop an exagerated posterior thoracic convexity (T-older people develop an exagerated posterior thoracic convexity-a kyphosis, due to atrophy of the intervertebral discs)

18. Central cord syndrome: (T/F)
a) Is more common in children than adults (F-central cord syndrome is more common in elderly patients)
b) The paresis affects the lower limbs more than the upper limbs (F-the opposite is true. The upper limbs are more affected than the lower limbs)
c) Characteristically has a fracture visible on plain x-rays

(F-there are no specific features on plain x-rays. Degenerative changes are often seen on the x-rays of elderly patients, but these are incidental findings)
d) Has a variable pattern of sensory deficit (T)

19. The following structures are clearly visible on a lateral cervical spine radiograph: (T/F)
a) Vertebral bodies (T)
b) Spinous processes (T)
c) Transverse processes (F-transverse processes are visible on AP radiographs)
d) Facet joints (T)

20. Spinal cord injury without radiographic injury (SCIWORA): (T/F)
a) Can be caused by epidural haematoma (T)
b) Only occurs in children (F-although unusual, SCIWORA does occur in adults)
c) Has a characteristic pattern of neurological deficit (F-the neurological features, if any, are variable)
d) Can be caused by ligamentous instability (T)

www.ingramcontent.com/pod-product-compliance
Lightning Source LLC
Chambersburg PA
CBHW061509180526
45171CB00001B/96